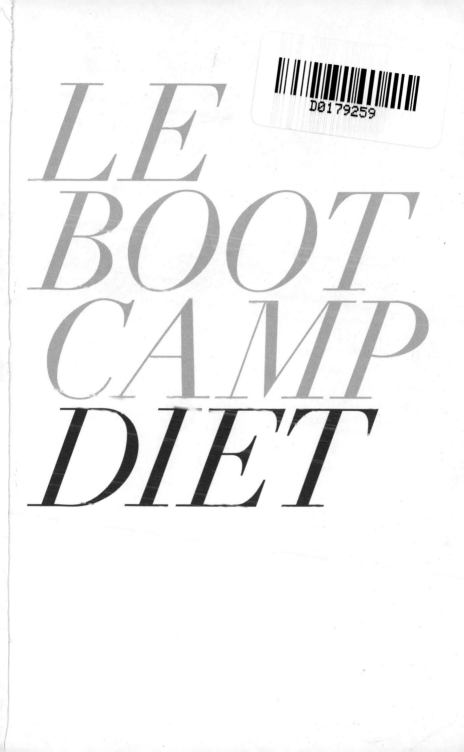

LE
BOOT
CAMP
DIET

To my son, Baptiste, for his motto:
"If there is no solution there is no problem."
So true.

LE BOOT CAMP DIET

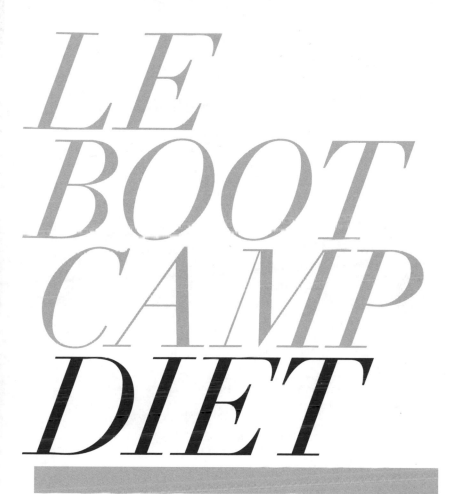

EAT WELL
LOSE WEIGHT NOW
KEEP IT OFF FOREVER

VALÉRIE ORSONI

Publishing Director:
Jane O'Shea
Creative Director:
Helen Lewis
Editor and Project Manager:
Charlotte Coleman-Smith
Design and Art Direction:
Untitled
Photographer Rita Platts
Production Director:
Vincent Smith
Production Controller:
Emily Noto

Back jacket photograph
© Mikel Healey
Inside back jacket
photograph © Aaron
Blumenshine Photography

First published in 2015 by
Quadrille Publishing Ltd
Pentagon House
52–54 Southwark Street
London SE1 1UN

www.quadrille.co.uk
Text © 2015 Valérie Orsoni

Design and layout
© 2015 Quadrille
Publishing Limited

Reprinted in 2014
10 9 8 7 6 5 4 3 2

Cataloguing in Publication
data: a catalogue record
for this book is available
from the British Library.

ISBN 978-1-84949-530-1
Printed in the UK

CONTENTS

INTRODUCTION

FOUR PHASES
FOUR PILLARS
FOUR PLEDGES
FOUR PRINCIPLES

Let me introduce myself.

I am a woman just like you.
I have battled with weight issues and frustrating fad diets for years.
I do not believe in a life of deprivation and yo-yo dieting

After trying more than 40 diets – on my own (Cabbage Soup, The Prehistoric); with my family (Pineapple, Low-calorie, Hyper-protein) or alongside friends (Dissociated, Fasting, High-protein); after losing and regaining weight that eventually burst the seams of my jeans; after feeling taunted by so many failures and demoralised when I looked at myself in the mirror, I woke up one morning and decided that I had simply had enough!

Tired of nonsensical approaches, ranging from terribly restrictive menus to dangerously protein-rich diets, I decided to educate myself in order to understand my excess weight better and attack it intelligently.

To do this, I joined forces with my father, who was also overweight at the time. Together, we committed to maintaining a gourmet approach no matter what (we loved eating too much to deprive ourselves continuously, and yes, we are French, or Corsican, rather).

It may seem like something from the Stone Age, but our research led us to the library – this was well before the Internet had made its appearance in our homes. There, we devoured books on nutrition, fitness – even psychology! Gradually, we began to gather together and put to the test those concepts which seemed logical and healthy. Along the way we came to terms with the fact that if it had taken us years to gain weight, it would be unreasonable to attempt to lose it all in two weeks via tasteless meals and mono diets.

The results? After one year of a patchwork approach which brought together everything that worked from each diet we researched, we had achieved our ideal weight, without any suffering or deprivation.

And then? My friends began asking for my help to get healthy and slim. I was burning out in a fast-paced, corporate job at the time. So I decided to give greater meaning to my life and share this knowledge with millions of women like myself, who were on the verge of giving up. Thus was born LeBootCamp.com.

Not being a doctor myself, I was soon facing criticism from those medical professionals who promote diet pills and supplements. Despite giving watertight explanations for the concepts I had proven, the programme's blatant success appeared to mean very little when not dressed in medical jargon. Clearly, it was too late in life to go to medical school, so, I surrounded myself with dozens of experts who knew more than me: physicians, dietitians, scientists, Olympic athletes, nutritionists and psychologists, in order to test out my theories.

Unlike those 'miracle diets' which have remained unchanged since the Seventies, LeBootCamp Diet evolves constantly, embracing new, medical and scientific discoveries and ensuring that its techniques remain effective over the long term. We are diligent in our work: indeed, we require that any new concept absorbed into LeBootCamp Diet be supported by at least five double-blind medical studies on a representative sample (a sample of five people is not valid!), according to serious and verifiable protocols.

We conducted a study to monitor 800 women who followed LeBootCamp programme over a period of six months. The sample was divided into two groups of 400: the first group for a cholesterol study and the second group for a glycaemia control study. After one month on the LeBootCamp programme, the average weight loss for both groups – besides improvements in glycaemia control and cholesterol levels – was 6kg. And after six months, the average weight lost and never regained, rose to 13kg.

And men?

Although I initially started my programme catering only to the needs of women, I soon realised that BootCampers®' male partners also liked the recipes, the stress-reduction exercises and our fitness routines.

So, don't hesitate to share this book with your boyfriend, male friend or partner. Enrol them in your programme. Make them taste your new dishes; invite them to cook with (and for!) you. Very soon, you will have a slimmer partner – and your most loyal supporter!

VALÉRIE ORSONI, San Francisco, January 2015

FOUR PHASES

DETOX
To cleanse your body

ATTACK
To lose weight

BOOSTER
To speed up the process!

MAINTENANCE
To ensure you never
regain lost weight

1   DETOX

The foundation of the programme. A two-week phase, where my top 10 detoxifying foods are incorporated into balanced menus designed to nourish your body with antioxidants, eliminate toxins and give you more energy.

WHAT YOU ACHIEVE First pounds are shed quickly, energy is regained, skin is glowing.

KEY CONCEPT Detoxification.

2   ATTACK

Now that your body has been cleansed and the first few pounds have gone, you are ready to attack the stubborn weight that remains and reduce cellulite. This second phase lasts as long as it takes to lose 75 per cent of the weight you need to shed. With my guidance, you will establish healthy life habits and learn how to balance your daily meals.

A Turbo Detox Day (TD Day) is featured every week to promote the elimination of toxins and enhance weight loss. You will gradually integrate new foods and flavours into delicious, light recipes. During ATTACK you will find weight loss effective and motivating, allowing you to reach your ideal weight with ease.

WHAT YOU ACHIEVE Stubborn pounds are targeted, attacked and eliminated; you lose 75 per cent of the weight you want to shed; cellulite is greatly reduced; body is toned.

KEY CONCEPTS Glycaemic load and its impact on weight loss. Additionally, during this phase I will introduce you to the concept of benchmarking, a strategy that ensures you continue to lose weight as you go along. You'll learn how to transform those dreaded 'plateaus' into secure milestones, each one a personal victory.

3   BOOSTER

This enhancing routine lasts seven days and recurs several times throughout the programme. You should repeat it every time you reach the end of a benchmark during the ATTACK phase or, once you are in the MAINTENANCE phase, whenever you feel the need to renew yourself; for example, after a hen weekend, after a holiday where the food was irresistible, after a period of intense stress at work, or if you are keen to achieve a flatter stomach.

Throughout this short interval, we abstain from meat, dairy, yeast, gluten and alcohol in order truly to support the detoxifying functions of our body.

> **WHAT YOU ACHIEVE** A cleansed body more able to lose pounds quickly and a flat abdomen.

> **KEY CONCEPTS** Extreme cleansing and the yeast connection.

4   MAINTENANCE

This last phase is unlimited. With the help of this book, and also with our Facebook page (www.facebook.com/groups/lebootcampdiet) and its active community; our website (LeBootCamp.com); our Twitter (twitter.com/lebootcamp) and Instagram (@valerieorsoni) feeds, you will learn to create balanced menus for yourself as well as handle various life challenges: restaurants, parties, social engagements, travelling and so on.

Once you have shed your final pounds, your weight will naturally stabilise. Physical activity will become an integral part of your daily life as you tone those last few stubborn areas. By then you will know how to avoid nutritional pitfalls and the trap of fad diets. You will be ready to pursue your healthy journey independently and with confidence and will never regain your lost weight!

> **WHAT YOU ACHIEVE** Your ideal weight is maintained and your energy levels are high. You love your body!

> **KEY CONCEPTS** Alkaline-balancing to support a healthy life and keep the pounds off.

FOUR PILLARS

1   GOURMET NUTRITION

Some eat to live. I live to eat, and personally, I am convinced that there is nothing worse than a life governed by deprivation and tasteless meals. Yes, I promise you, we can live a healthy, long life AND enjoy delicious foods from all food groups.

Back when I was a child growing up in France, my dad was a chef and I had the privilege of being introduced to a cuisine rich in diversity that shaped my tastebuds – though, I must admit, there are foods I cannot even imagine myself eating anymore (think snails or tripe). Let's go back to our roots, when we truly enjoyed everything that nature has to offer. There are no forbidden foods in my programme!

Let's face it, we all have hectic lives and rarely use our gym membership (that is, if we can afford one in the first place). We need to reclaim our birthright and rediscover what our bodies were designed to do, when we were fit and trim without the gym. There is a direct correlation between the advent of gyms, food labels and new diets; and obesity, and it is not what we think. The obesity epidemic did not, in fact, give rise to these. Shockingly, it is the reverse. By infantilising society, these familiar props of modern life have only worsened the problem.

In truth, in our most natural state, we shouldn't have to suffer, military-style, to get in shape, or force ourselves to break into a sweat for hours at the gym. This is precisely what the fitness aspect of my programme is about: getting your heart pumping and your muscles moving without too much effort – the 'in-shape-no-sweat' approach. Follow my '25th-hour' exercises (pages 46 –49) and you'll see how easy it is to fit exercise into an already busy day.

3   MOTIVATION

Knowing what's right is not enough. The proof? Hundreds of books have been published on health and dieting by doctors, gurus, nutritionists, nurses, dietitians and coaches – yet still, nobody has succeeded in reducing the obesity epidemic.

On the other hand, learning what works one day at a time, whilst taking on board small but effective new techniques, is the surest path to a slimmer you. A study conducted by Berkeley University, in California, proved this fact beyond any doubt. Two groups of individuals were observed over the course of 18 months: the first one was given all the instructions to lose weight in one 'sitting', while the second was given one element per day for 90 days. After 18 months the second group had lost twice as much weight and kept it off for longer than the first group.

This is why I can guarantee that, if you follow my programme, we will win the fight against those stubborn pounds one day at a time, step by step, until we reach your perfect weight. For the days when you feel down, when 'motivation' is a meaningless word to you, when diet saboteurs challenge your grit, I will arm you with proven techniques to help you stay on track, no matter what.

Despite multiple studies linking stress to obesity, the connection is commonly overlooked and causes many diets to fail. Since a happy dieter is a successful dieter, I offer you a guilt-free approach, based on proven strategies, which will help you reclaim your inner peace and lessen your stress levels. This will, in turn, reduce your cortisol levels, improve the quality of your sleep and trim down belly fat. Focused exercise, abdominal breathing, visualisation techniques and my own, widely-respected motivational methodologies will bring your body and mind into closer harmony. Your energy will soar.

FOUR PLEDGES

1   ETHICS

Because of my own negative experience with fad diets and simply because of the way I am wired, my approach is underpinned by the highest level of respect for you. You can trust that I abide by a strict code of ethics, in that everything I share with you is based on solid medical and scientific foundations. I've tried to present these principles in a fun way, to make them easier to understand and implement in your everyday life.

2   HEALTH

Everything we do in life should have a positive impact on our health and well-being. That's why my most fundamental objective is to enhance your fitness and vitality. After risking my own health with dangerous diets, I am now totally committed to a healthy lifestyle. And this is what I share with you in my programme, firm in the belief that a healthy body is one that sheds kilos faster and does not regain lost weight.

3   QUALITY

I'll be brief: quality goes hand-in-hand with the highest standards of ethics and health; I will never compromise these standards. I am dedicated to making sure that the products and services I present to you are always of the highest degree of excellence. Enough said.

4   INNOVATION

Boredom and monotony are largely responsible when it comes to diet failures. Just take one look at how short-lived high-protein and mono diets turn out to be. I love exploring new foods, new concepts or new fitness trends, which keep me on my toes, always on the look-out. Count on me for sharing new products and ideas with you that will make your weight-loss journey easier and more fun.

FOUR PRINCIPLES

1 NO FORBIDDEN FOOD GROUPS

FACT Banning certain foods leads to yo-yo dieting.

Because I have experienced first-hand what happens when you're deprived of certain foods, I made a promise to myself never, ever to inflict such extreme measures on my body again. Besides being unhealthy, this deprivation leads to obsessive-compulsive behaviours, which, in turn, trigger 'yo-yo' dieting (lose weight, regain more, lose more, regain more, and so on).

Hence, no food group is banned from my diet. Some foods are evidently healthier than others – I recommend you avoid unnecessary toxins by always eating organic – and we will focus on them.

2   BODY-CLEANSING

FACT A clean body is a lean body. A clean body supports rapid, healthy weight loss.

Our body certainly has the right equipment to rid itself of the toxins we produce, ingest, inhale, or absorb through our skin. However, in our fast-paced world, with increased environmental pollution, the rise of pesticides and other chemicals in our food chain, and the extremely high levels of stress we face, our body is under too much strain for its basic detoxification functions to be sufficient. Hence a DETOX phase, a Turbo Detox Day (TD Day), and a recurring BOOSTER phase to support our body's cleansing ability.

3   ALKALINE-BALANCING

FACT An acidic body is a tired and vulnerable body.
An alkaline body is an energetic and healthy body.

We measure the acidity level of our system using pH-grading, aiming for a perfect urine pH of seven (that of pure water) to best support all our bodily functions. Most importantly the rate of our weight loss improves when our body has the perfect alkaline-acid balance.

4   SUGAR-MANAGEMENT

FACT We all consume too much refined sugar

A direct link has been established between the rise in obesity and the dramatic rise in sugar consumption (from 4.5kg per person per year in 1815, to 54kg in 2000). On top of pure sugar, we consume way too many high-glycaemic foods, which turn our body into fat-storing machines. Together we will learn how to enjoy the sweetness in life without jeopardising our weight-loss efforts.

Does my approach work?

Don't take my word for it! BootCampers from around the world have endorsed it. Check out their testimonials here: www.lebootcamp.com/en/success/view.

Before letting you dive into the last diet of your life, let me also share with you the story of Patricia, my first ever weight-loss client. It was exactly one week after Thanksgiving 2003 when I launched my first online, weight-loss coaching website. As much as I had mastered subjects like nutrition, fitness and coaching, I was a total beginner when it came to business: I had no business plan, no business bank account, nor any idea of the price at which I would set my services. Let's face it: I had launched my business without thinking at all about its structure – so full of joy and hope was I at the prospect of helping other women around the world reach their ideal weight!

I was riding the Caltrain, which links San Francisco to the suburbs. A rather plump woman next to me struck up conversation (in the USA people tend to chat with strangers rather easily).

"Gosh, you're lucky to be so skinny!" she said. "Mother Nature has been kind to you. You look amazing!" To which I replied, "Mother Nature is kind only if you help her – trust me, I waged a battle against unwanted pounds for as long as I can remember; until I worked out a healthy strategy to get the results I'd wanted for so long. Now, I am actually launching my very own, healthy programme online."

"What a great idea!" she exclaimed. "How much does it cost and when can I get started?" This marked the beginning of a great adventure during which Patricia lost 20kg, which she never regained.

So, are you ready? Great! To help you get started, here are 10 steps I recommend you follow before embarking on phase one of my programme: namely, DETOX.

TOP 10 PRE-DETOX STEPS

1 Decide on your weight-loss goal: write it on a Post-it that you place on the mirror in your bathroom as a constant reminder.

2 Involve your friends: sharing a goal means being accountable. Social networks make your life easier when it comes to finding support. Sign up your friends in your fight against those unwanted pounds.

3 Decide on the start date: this is vital! By consciously choosing your first day you will have taken the step that will guarantee that you get started.

4 Grocery shopping: stock up on everything you will need for the first week (go to p. 58 to check out the menus and draw up your shopping list).

5 Get rid of temptations: give away everything you won't be eating during the DETOX and BOOSTER phases.

6 Buy your equipment: to get the most out of my programme you will need a juicer, a blender, a pedometer (or an app on your smartphone that counts steps and distance) and a pair of well-fitting walking shoes. If you don't have everything right away, don't fret! For instance, if you don't have a juicer then you can mix your fruits/veggies in a blender and strain the juice with a piece of muslin.

7 Walk: start walking 30 minutes every single morning before your breakfast – but after your morning drinks: lemon, green tea and Sobacha (p. 71). Get your heart pumping!

8 Pre-detox: not quite ready to start today? No problem! Get set right now by doing a few things to make sure you don't keep delaying the true start. Get going by eliminating red meat and dairy from your daily meals.

9 Drink water: drink at least eight glasses of water each day. Keep in mind that hydration needs vary from person to person. The best way to determine if you should drink more is to look at the colour of your urine: if it is dark yellow it means you aren't drinking enough; if it's is clear, you are already doing a great job.

10 Weigh yourself! Do this right now, and then once a week, if that works for you. Once you begin the DETOX diet, weigh yourself daily or at least every other day. (I like a daily weigh-in to stay on track). Record your starting weight on 'Your weight-loss progress page' (p. 244).

What is my ideal weight?

All weight-loss experts (me included) have tried to come up with a perfect formula. Even if it is important to know how to calculate one's ideal weight (because this will be our target), you should remember that there is no perfect solution, no magic number.

Indeed, amongst all the formulae dreamed up by doctors, online calculators and insurance companies (which very often add two to 10kg to what we consider our sexy, ideal weight), it is extremely difficult to know whom to trust, especially when we are also being bombarded with images of extremely skinny models in women's magazines.

So how can we evaluate our ideal weight? Start by using the Creff formula, which calculates your ideal weight (in kg) purely from a health perspective. This formula corrects the more famous Lorentz formula as it brings in two further considerations: age and morphology.

Have you ever heard someone say, "I can never be skinny because I have big bones"? Well, with the Creff formula, the size of your bones is taken into consideration. In terms of morphology, for an individual with a slight frame, 10 per cent is subtracted from the weight calculated for an average person. Conversely, for someone with a large morphology, 10 per cent is added to the average ideal weight.

To determine if you are small, average, or broad, place the middle finger and thumb of your right hand around your left wrist:

SMALL your thumb slightly overlaps your middle finger

AVERAGE your thumb and finger just touch

BROAD your thumb and finger don't even touch

CREFF FORMULA

Small morphology:

[(height in centimetres) − 100 + (age in years/10)] x 0.9 x 0.9

Average morphology:

[(height in centimetres) − 100 + (age in years/10)] x 0.9

Broad morphology:

[(height in centimetres) − 100 + (age in years/10)] x 0.9 x 1.1

NOTE this formula is only one indication of your health. It is totally possible that your perceived ideal weight (the one at which you feel proud of yourself in your bikini) is under (rarely over) this number. For example, my ideal weight is 3.5kg under the weight determined by the Creff formula.

It is essential to keep in mind that your ideal weight is the one you can maintain without depriving yourself and without intense efforts. For instance, I am 157cm tall. If I weigh 48kg, I look hot on TV and in a bikini, but it is extremely hard for me to maintain this weight and I need truly to deprive myself to stay at that level. At 48kg, I get ill easily and my energy levels are low. Now, if I use the Creff Formula my ideal weight is 55kg, but then I feel heavy and sluggish − far from the energetic bunny I have become famous for being. However, when I am 52kg, I am generally at the top of my game, energy-wise, and almost never sick.

Now is your turn to determine your ideal weight, using the Creff Formula to start with, before comparing it with where you feel at your best. This will be your personal 'cruising weight', and the one we will be aiming to reach and maintain.

DETOX

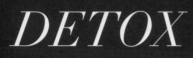

GOAL

Detox your lifestyle
and reset your body
to lose your first
pounds rapidly

DETOX

FACT

- Stress is fattening; the accumulation of toxins stemming from our lifestyle, environment and food prevents us from losing weight.

Rules of the DETOX phase

- We detox our body with **FIVE** detox foods per day. It is very important that even if you modify the menus, you stick to this magic number.
- We drink Sobacha® every morning, plus three cups throughout the day.
- We drink lemon juice with water every morning.
- We avoid red meat, cow dairy, eggs, rich sauces, sugar products, heavy foods, gluten, yeast and alcohol, all of which can overload our system in different ways.
- We do five '25th-hour' exercises per day.
- We manage our stress with abdominal breathing exercises.

These first 14 days of my programme are critical to the success of my weight-loss strategy. That is why I urge you *not* to skip directly to the second phase (I know some might be tempted). Everything has been designed to put you on the right track to a slimmer you. Thousands of women have followed my programme, and it's thanks to their valuable feedback that I have been able to devise and adapt this first, vital phase.

I must warn you right away: these two weeks won't be the easiest in my plan. But rest assured, they remain true to my philosophy of yummy nutrition and easy fitness. If you're feeling apprehensive, just project yourself to the place, two weeks from now, when you'll be feeling the full effects of this detox: your first few pounds will have vanished, leaving you feeling lighter, more energetic and highly motivated!

WHAT IS A DETOX?

In the strict sense of the word, detoxification means helping our body get rid of addictive or toxic substances.

The word 'detox' appeared for the first time in 1973, in an American women's magazine – a time when our world had started spinning faster and our days were becoming more hectic. Incidentally, that is when we also noticed a spike in weight curves in the Western world.

Forty years later, this term has broadened to cover a vast range of therapies, including the rehab of substance-abuse addicts; therapeutic nutrition retreats designed to flush toxins out of the system, and simple, healthy-living detox camps.

WHY DO TOXINS PREVENT ME FROM LOSING WEIGHT?

A toxin is a substance that our body does not need and which requires energy to be eliminated. Even some elements vital to our survival can become toxic in large quantities. As my grandmother used to say, "Too much of a good thing can be bad!"

Not only are we surrounded by toxins – bacteria, parasites, viruses, pesticides, pollution and chemical products (including paraben-loaded beauty products) – but we also directly ingest a large portion of toxins via the food we eat. Thus, food becomes our number-one source of toxins! Remember that toxins can be carcinogenic, and 'carcinogenic' means 'can cause cancer'.

The beauty of the detox process is that food, our first source of toxicity, is also the best and easiest way to clean up our body. What's more, weight loss will automatically begin as you start to detox!

How so? Our body handles toxic aggressions by encapsulating toxins in fat cells; hence, the more toxins we carry, the larger our fat cells become (the actual number of fat cells never changes). The detoxification process helps reduce the area of fat mass where these fat-soluble toxins are stored.

Here's the equation: when we reduce the toxin content in our body we reduce the quantity of fat that is stored. Then we enter a virtuous circle where we have fewer toxins to store and, therefore, less fat required to store them.

HOW DOES THE BODY ELIMINATE TOXINS NATURALLY?

The word 'detox', is, unfortunately, often misused by charlatans around the world. It greatly antagonises some doctors, who refuse even to acknowledge that the concept exists. They argue that the body is naturally equipped to clean itself through its hepatic and kidney functions and that detox programmes serve no purpose.

However, those old-school doctors might as well go back to ... school! You only need to look at an alcoholic's liver or the lungs of a heavy-smoker to realise that even our perfectly programmed body has its limits when it comes to getting rid of toxins. Yet there's just no need for expensive (and, sometimes, dangerous) detox products or programmes. My DETOX phase is simple, proven, affordable – and it will help you shed your unwanted pounds. Trust your coach!

The body has developed two ways of eliminating toxins:

1 Internal: our body has an extraordinarily complex system that modifies, attacks and eliminates threats to our health. For hundreds of thousands of years our body has been reliant upon this system. Unfortunately for us, with the drastic increase in the number of toxic products we are now exposed to, and their poor quality, our liver, stomach, immune system, kidneys and lungs can't cope with the load any more. So, we need to support our organs by way of a complete detox programme.

2 External: thanks to the sweat glands in the skin, it can also help us eliminate a large quantity of toxins. Supporting this function is very easy: you need to sweat! Either by exercising, or – and this is even more efficient – by sitting in a steam room or sauna for a prescribed time.

> **NOTE** Never stay longer than 20 minutes in a sauna and *never* use them as an alternative to exercise or a healthy diet.

In our daily life, we can point the finger at three major sources of toxins that are responsible, among other things, for our extra weight: food, stress and external pollutants. Together, we shall take action against those three culprits.

Toxic diets

Extreme diets can actually be a source of toxins. If you have ever followed a high-protein diet, you have most likely regained all the weight you lost; you might also remember that during this diet your skin looked dull, your breath was terrible, your energy low, your mood swings extreme and your headaches frequent. Nutritionist associations and some followers of high-protein diets have even reported kidney failure as a direct result of the diet.

Why? Because your body is not equipped to eliminate the excessive amount of protein residues (ketone bodies) generated when exposed to a radical protein intake. These residues are toxins which have to be eliminated through our kidneys. This is why you have to drink a lot of water on a high-protein diet (which I, therefore, cannot advise you to follow!).

The same toxic punishment results if you follow a mono diet like the Cabbage Soup Diet, the Pineapple Diet or the Lemon Juice/Cayenne Pepper Diet.

And if you think that fasting will solve the problem – you are totally mistaken! In fact, pushed outside its healthy comfort zone our fasting body will get its energy from fat stores and from our muscle mass (not from our digestive tract or glycogen reserves as in a normal, balanced diet). This leads to a high production of waste, causing an increase of the toxin levels in the body.

1 FOOD

Our refined modern diet is often characterised by excessive protein and a deficient fibre content, with too much saturated fat, too much sugar and too much sodium (that's your kitchen salt).

Over 2,800 substances (preservatives, artificial colours, sweeteners) are used by the food industry to improve taste, texture, colour and the shelf-life of products. The problem is that they often increase the toxin levels in our body. Add to these the pesticides used to grow your food and we get an explosive mix of toxins that our body struggles to excrete, leaving it exhausted (one of the reasons you're feeling so tired!).

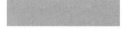

Top five toxins in our food

1 Mercury from large, carnivorous fish

I love fish, as they are rich in healthy fats (those famous omega-3s, said to boost brain function) and lean protein.

Fish possess precious nutritional qualities. The problem is that they are also contaminated by environmental pollutants like dioxins, methylmercury, PCBs (polychlorinated byphenols), and so on. Mercury can mainly be found in fat fish like tuna and the flesh of other wild predators in the fish family. Because they are so high up the food chain, larger fish accumulate more of those pollutants by eating smaller fish.

Chronic exposure to mercury has been proven to have terrible health consequences, notably for our nervous system, leading to tingling in the limbs, blurred vision, hearing problems and cognitive deficiencies. Exposure to methylmercury while pregnant can also trigger neurological developmental delays and growth issues in the foetus. Furthermore, methylmercury can also have an adverse impact on our digestive system and kidneys.

For these reasons, I advise you to limit yourself to small fish like anchovies and sardines; wild fish from protected places like Alaska (although they will still contain some environmental toxins, owing to water flowing freely around the globe); or organically farmed fish. I really insist on organic fish-farming as non-organic fish farms frequently use food with questionable ingredients, some of them very toxic. Don't take my word for it, just go and visit one!

2 Pesticides and chemical treatments used in agriculture

Some environmental toxins, like chemical fertilisers, pesticides, fungicides and other synthetic products used by the agriculture industry, can be found in the fruits and vegetables you buy at your favourite market. The problem with these toxic elements is that, once ingested, they can mimic our 'body messengers', or hormones. That is why pesticides are often called 'endocrine disruptors'. Some pesticides are capable of mimicking the effects of oestrogens – hormones produced naturally by our body – and can cause numerous illnesses such as obesity, diabetes and cardiovascular diseases. Over-exposure to oestrogens has also been proven to increase the risk of breast cancer. Indeed, by affecting our endocrine system, those pesticides can affect the actions of neurotransmitters (chemical messengers, such as serotonin) and have a negative impact on our metabolism.

FACT The Golden Delicious apple receives 32 chemical treatments from the time of pollination until its arrival on your plate. Go organic!

3 High-fructose corn syrup (HFCS)

The term 'fructose syrup' makes us think of ordinary white sugar, in its liquid form. However, high-fructose syrup is actually far from natural and is becoming increasingly common in our food. You may well be consuming it without even knowing. Check the labels on your biscuits, sweets and ready meals. Even innocent-looking crackers may contain it. So, what is it?

This syrup, invented in 1957, is made primarily from corn starch. Its low cost – three times less expensive than sugar – together with its superior sweetening and taste-enhancement properties, make it a perfect candidate for the manufacturing of low-priced sweets and biscuits. It's now ubiquitous on supermarket shelves and is slowly but surely replacing the traditional sucrose (ordinary white sugar) in processed foods.

Replacing sucrose with high-fructose corn syrup has little or no impact on taste. However, the effect of HFCS on our hormonal functions is an invisible menace.

But why, you might wonder, is fructose a 'good' sugar when present in fruit, but not when it is found in HFCS? Fructose in fruits is ok because it is combined with fibre, water and other ingredients. Isolated from fibre (which slows down the digestion of sugar) and consumed in large quantities, HFCS will increase our triglyceride (fat) and cholesterol lovels, leading to an over storage of fat and excess weight.

I'm sure you get the picture: in order to remain slim or to lose weight, you must become an educated shopper and always read food labels. If you see HFCS, fructose/glucose sugar, fructose/glucose syrup, corn sugar, or corn syrup on the label, don't buy it!

4   Artificial sweeteners

The black sheep of the dieting world, I am deeply convinced, is the artificial sweetener. Official studies and meta-studies prove that it is largely responsible for the obesity epidemic and for the fact that the vast majority of overweight individuals find it hard to lose weight.

These sweeteners have been invading our food for decades. With a sweetening power equal or superior to that of regular white sugar, artificial sweeteners don't contain any calories. What a miracle! Finally to be able to consume sweet foods without putting on weight – who hasn't dreamt of it? So, what's the catch?

Researchers have found that if we trick our brain into thinking that we are eating something sweet without the intake of calories our body is expecting, the sweet craving is exacerbated. A study by Irish researchers looking at the impact of diet drinks on the eating habits of ordinary people (not athletes) proved this beyond doubt. They concluded that diet drinks and foods blur our ability to sense hunger.

> **FACT** Diet foods can be a trap. They are expensive, and can never replace a balanced diet.

Let's look at the most readily available sweeteners on the market and you'll see that some represent a far healthier choice than others:

- **Acesulfame K:** this synthetic sweetener has a sweetening power 200 times stronger than that of regular sugar, but contains zero calories. It is highly resistant to heat, so can be used for baking. However, it is, literally, too good to be true as it can't be metabolised by the body. To be avoided.

- **Aspartame:** this artificial sweetener, also called E951, was created in 1965 and is 200 times sweeter than sugar. Since its launch on the US market in 1974, it has caused a great deal of controversy but, owing to a very powerful lobby, it has succeeded in remaining in our food. It can now be found in almost all 'diet' or 'light' yogurts, biscuits, sweets, chewing gums and ice-creams.

  NOTE In Dec 2013 the European Food Safety Authority published a report claiming that aspartame is safe and poses no threat to our health.

It is interesting to note that in the USA this sweetener is not recommended for pregnant women or diabetics – but this is not the case in France, Italy or the UK. However, even though aspartame is calorie-free, it still affects your blood-sugar levels just like white sugar would, by stimulating the pancreas to produce insulin. This reaction causes the body to store more of the 'real' food you've eaten, in the form of fat.

That's why even low-calorie fizzy drinks (very likely to be sweetened with aspartame), transform you into a fat-storing machine. What's more, if the fizzy drink is served freezing cold, as is commonly the case, your appetite will be further intensified and you will most likely order more food. In terms of drinks, you are always better off with regular water or green tea (which has a low caffeine content).

- **Erythritol:** another polyol. Though discovered in 1874, it took some years before this was used by the food industry. Erythritol is a natural sweetener found in fruits, fermented foods and soy sauce. It has a slightly higher sweetening power than sugar, with two advantages: it does not cause cavities and contains zero calories. So far, no study has ever shown its danger to our health.

Effects of aspartame on appetite

The impact of aspartame on weight gain has been proven numerous times, but one of my favourite studies is the famous one conducted by Dr Katherine Appleton, of Queen's University, Belfast:

Three runners are given a bottle of liquid to drink, without knowing what it is.

The first bottle contains water, the second one contains a fizzy drink sweetened with ordinary sugar, and the third bottle contains a diet drink sweetened with aspartame.

After each runner has drunk her bottle, she is made to run for 20 minutes.

After the run each participant is presented with an identical meal with one instruction: stop eating when you aren't hungry any more.

This experiment is repeated over the course of 10 years, and the same result is noted each time: the runners eating more are always the ones who initially consumed the diet drink. On average, they take in an average of 150 extra calories at each meal.

Despite Katherine Appleton's research, manufacturers of diet drinks consistently deny that their products cause an increased feeling of hunger.

But if it's true that drinking a diet soda sweetened with aspartame before a meal increases your food intake by 150 calories, as Dr Appleton concluded, after 50 days this will lead to a weight gain of around 1kg (since you need approximately 7,500 extra calories to make 1kg of fat).

Scary!

- **Fructose:** this natural fruit sugar has the lowest glycaemic index amongst all the sweeteners and has long been recommended to diabetics as a sugar substitute. However, after more research, we know that although fructose does not cause a rise in blood sugar, it does trigger an increase in triglyceride levels (fat levels in the blood). So, it's fine to consume fructose in its natural form (as the fibre contained in fruit prevents the triglyceride level increase) but it should never be used as a sweetener. To be avoided.

- **Maltitol:** this sweetener is responsible for that intense sense of freshness you get from some foods (notably chewing gums). Maltitol is a polyol, or sugar alcohol, and one of the rare sweeteners to be authorised for diabetics because it does not affect blood sugar. It is derived from maltose (found in starch) and can have laxative effects in large quantities. Unlike some other sweeteners it is non cavity-forming and should be chosen over aspartame. It's not calorie-free, though: it contains 2.4 calories per gram (as opposed to four calories per gram for sucrose).

- **Saccharine:** the dinosaur of all artificial sweeteners! Created in 1879, it has a very high sweetening power (300 to 400 times that of regular sugar), zero calories and leaves a strong metallic taste in the mouth. Saccharine withstands heat and has a long shelf life, so is now used as a stabiliser in combination with other sweeteners.

- **Stevia:** consumed in Japan since the Fifties, this now represents over 75 per cent of the sweeteners sold in this country. Although no study proving any health dangers has ever been published, it still took years for other countries to authorise stevia as a food supplement. As of 2014, it can be found in all Western countries. Stevia is a herbaceous plant from the Asteraceae family. Its leaves, dried and crushed, have a very sweet taste and have been used for thousands of years in South America and China. It has zero calories and a sweetening power 150 to 300 higher than that of sugar. You can use stevia for baking, but not for making jams as it cannot be heated above 220°C. Stevia also lowers blood-sugar levels, reduces blood pressure and is a natural, mild diuretic. Since it does not increase blood sugar it is a natural ally for diabetics. Recommended until proven otherwise.

- **Sucralose:** found everywhere (except France where it was banned in 2012) and made from ordinary white sugar (sucrose). It has a high sweetening power with zero calories. Following a few studies pointing out potential dangers, it has suffered from rather bad press. However, no serious double-blind study has been conducted long enough to gauge whether or not sucralose has any negative impact on health. Until there is evidence to the contrary, I avoid using it on a regular basis (but if I run out of stevia this sweetener would be my second choice).

• **Xylitol:** this polyol is extracted from the bark of the birch tree. Often sold in powder form, xylitol has the same sweetening power and the same taste as ordinary white sugar but has half the calories. It has two main advantages: it protects our teeth by preventing the fermentation of bacteria and also remineralises them, a property that none of the other polyols have.

5   Other additives: artificial colourings, flavour enhancers and preservatives

We have been using additives since the dawn of time (well, almost) to improve taste, texture, colour and the shelf-life of food. Romans used saltpetre (or potassium nitrate), Egyptians used food colourings and, towards the end of the nineteenth century, the first chemical leavening agent was created. As we've discussed, while many of these have huge advantages, they also increase the toxin levels in our body, which can lead to weight gain.

The biggest culprit is MSG (monosodium glutamate; code name E621 and also known as glutamate, sodium glutamate, glutamic acid, monopotassium glutamate, GMS and MSG). It is truly ubiquitous and can be found in chips, 'homemade' soups, sweets and in almost all ready meals. However, not only does MSG contain nothing good for our body, it also increases our appetite, thus making us overeat.

> **FACT** 40 years ago, a neuroscientist, Dr John Olney, from the School of Medicine at the University of Saint Louis, Washington, predicted that if E621 was authorised, the world would face an obesity epidemic and a massive rise in Diabetes Type II.

It's simple: avoid all products containing MSG and you will have made one solid step towards easy weight loss!

Before moving on to the menus, I would like to discuss some other causes of toxicity, besides what we put on our plates: stress and external pollutants.

Cigarettes, alcohol and caffeine

Cigarettes: smoking poisons the body, causes grey skin tone, lower lung capacity, fatigue and deprives you of half your vitamin C. Passive smoking harms those around you. However, one cannot fight on all fronts simultaneously. So, choose your battles in an order that works for you: lose weight first, then stop smoking, or the reverse, but not both at the same time, or you run the risk of failure. If you do smoke, the menus at the end of this chapter will help balance this dangerous addiction by supporting your body's ability to eliminate toxins.

Alcohol: can actually be good for you in very small quantities – this is the famous 'French paradox'. It has been proven that its polyphenols can guard us against cardiovascular diseases. If you drink one glass of red wine per day (two per day for men; life is unfair!) consider yourself protected. Beyond this level, wine becomes toxic. So we will be abstaining during DETOX and BOOSTER but the rest of the time you are allowed your daily glass of red wine. Isn't life wonderful?

Caffeine: this is not a poison, but if you drink too much during the day, as with many other things, you can give yourself palpitations and sleepless nights. That said, serious studies indicate that one coffee a day (enjoyed at leisure) can bring several benefits: it keeps you alert and is packed with antioxidants. Some studies have found an association between coffee consumption and decreased overall mortality as well as cardiovascular mortality, although this may not hold true for younger people who drink large amounts of coffee.

If you plan on drinking one or two small cups of coffee, may I suggest that you gradually replace those cups of coffee with tea or, even better, green tea?

Coffee is allowed in moderation during MAINTENANCE and ATTACK. However, it's best to abstain from it during DETOX and BOOSTER. That said, if refraining from your morning cuppa creates unnecessary and counterproductive stress, then have one cup, but no more.

2　STRESS

FACT Stress is fattening!

We cannot live without stress. It is essential to our survival and has been a companion both to human beings and animals since the dawn of time. So, despite so many of us complaining about it, it is stress we have to thank for our survival. It's responsible for the instinctive reflex that makes us jump out of the way of a speeding motorcycle or an aggressive dog. It is also stress that turns us into super-mums (and super-dads) when we need to juggle an already active life with a sick child and urgent projects to finish for yesterday. And, believe it or not, it is thanks to stress that we experience great happiness when we fall in love.

This tension sends a signal to our brain to help us adapt to stressful situations in daily life. However, when it comes to health and weight management, there is a major difference between acute stress (survival instinct) and chronic stress (also called oxidative stress), as the latter has been scientifically proven to cause weight gain.

Stress interacts directly with our levels of cortisol, a hormone produced by the kidneys, which affects the way in which our body manages our energy stores (i.e., stored fat). When stressed, our body produces more cortisol, which leads to an increase in blood-sugar levels.

A study conducted by Yale University showed that highly stressed women had higher cortisol levels (logical), and that their waist fat (also called toxic fat) was greater than that of the average woman under less stress. In addition, too much cortisol can lead to a depressive state which can, in turn, lead to snacking to compensate. Essentially, high levels of cortisol increase our attraction to sugar and bad fats (saturated fats). If you take note of what you crave when you're stressed, you will rarely notice a passion for cucumbers!

High levels of cortisol can also be blamed for increased storage of fat cells harbouring toxins. Eventually, they will also affect our thyroid, the gland responsible for the metabolism of all the cells in our body, thanks to the secretion of hormones (T3 and T4). If this gland stops working properly, the body can suffer a long-term lowering of its basal metabolism (the energy we need to stay alive). If we don't compensate for this by reducing our daily calorie intake or increasing our daily activity, we will end up storing more fat.

This is why, during the DETOX phase, we shall learn how to handle chronic stress more effectively (since we cannot totally eliminate it) and, as a result, reduce our cortisol and toxin levels considerably.

As we've seen, a 'lifestyle detox', which deals with stress as well as diet, is the key to jump-starting rapid weight loss.

HOW TO REDUCE NEGATIVE STRESS THAT FATTENS US UP

1   The problem: BEING REACHABLE 24/7!
Frequently consulting our Facebook feed, answering multiple text messages, picking up all incoming phone calls, reading news throughout the day, checking work emails on waking: being constantly connected and reachable is very stressful. These interruptions mean that we don't have one true moment to ourselves. To make things worse, all these activities are completely sedentary. We become overloaded; we power through the day, relying on adrenaline, which poisons our system and causes us to pile on the pounds.

The solution: A ONE-DAY NEWS AND SOCIAL MEDIA FAST
The world won't stop spinning because you don't read the news for 24 hours; you are not going to lose your Facebook friends if you don't update your status for one day. Choose, if possible, a day during the weekend so that you can take advantage of this electronic fast to go out and soak up some culture, try a new recipe, or meet with friends and go for a long walk in the countryside.

2   The problem: ENERGY VAMPIRES
Between a demanding boss who expects you to turn up to a meeting after work hours, when your youngest child leaves school at 3pm; a neighbour who listens to loud music at the crack of dawn; the girlfriend who asks, "Why do you bother dieting? You never succeed!", and the colleague who 'forgets' you are dieting and brings you

biscuits and sweets every single day, we are truly surrounded by what I call 'energy vampires'. They increase our level of stress and are responsible for some of our weight gain and our inability to lose those superfluous pounds.

The solution: IDENTIFY AND BANISH THOSE VAMPIRES!
Programme your toxic relation's emails to go directly into your junk folder. Invent a serious allergy to eggs or milk in order politely to excuse yourself from eating your co-worker's cakes and biscuits. Explain nicely to your boss that late meeting times can be scheduled earlier in the day. And if your neighbour listens to music at 6am, suggest he/she use it for exercise and then join in for the workout!

3   The problem: POOR BREATHING
Being stressed means breathing poorly. And breathing poorly means bloating. The equation is very simple!

How so? When we are stressed, we breathe in a shallow, or superficial way. This is because our diaphragm, which contracts and expands as we breathe, does not do its job properly any more. Our lungs don't inflate and deflate as they should, so we take in less oxygen. A tense diaphragm causes a compressed abdomen which can lead to intense abdominal pains and, more embarrassingly, gas. This is what gives us the dreaded and frustrating 'bloated' feeling.

To appreciate how far stress affects your tummy, just think: when you are stressed, have you noticed that you sometimes need to sigh or take in an extra-large deep breath? That doing so may even cause abdominal pain? That you feel a little bloated? The big culprit here really is the shallow breathing caused by intense stress.

The solution: LEARN HOW TO BREATHE FOR A FLAT TUMMY
Discover abdominal breathing by practising my favourite relaxation technique, 'Yoga Breathing'. This involves inflating your abdomen when you inhale through the nose (filling up deeply with air), and deflating it when you exhale through the mouth (breathing out deeply so your tummy goes flat). You don't need to force the move too much. Rather, follow your breath and let it circulate in a fluid manner.

Do this for two to three minutes every time you are stressed or, better yet, when you know that stress is likely to occur. Refer to the panel on page 42 for more of my favourite techniques.

Three stress-busting routines

Preparing for a stressful situation
1 Sit down with your back straight (against a wall). Imagine that you have a thread pulling you up from the top of your head.
2 Rest your left hand on your knee and shut your eyes.
3 Curl all the fingers of the right hand except your index finger and thumb.
4 With the index finger of your right hand close your left nostril and breathe in deeply; at the end of your inhalation close your right nostril with your thumb and release your index finger and breathe out through your left nostril.
5 Now breathe back in through your left nostril, close it gently, release your right nostril, then breathe out from the right and back in again.
6 Repeat the cycle calmly for five to 10 minutes. Try to make the exhalation twice as long as the inhalation.

Regaining your inner calm
1 Lie down on your back with your eyes closed and your legs bent, feet flat on the ground, hip-width apart.
2 Breathe in on a count of four.
3 Hold your breath for a few seconds.
4 Breathe out on a count of eight.
5 Repeat until you have regained your inner calm. You can take up to 16 counts to breathe out.

Fighting panic attacks and anxiety
1 Sit down with your back straight and your hands on your thighs.
2 Breathe in and out deeply and slowly.
3 Contracting your lower abdomen, breathe out little by little, around 10 or 20 times.
4 Inhale as if pronouncing the word 'so'.
5 Exhale with the sound of 'hum'. Continue for 10 to 15 minutes.

4   The problem: LACK OF SLEEP

You know this one already: we sleep poorly when we are under pressure. Studies prove that in our fast-paced society we sleep less and less, and that this lack of sleep can be linked to:

- Greater difficulty in losing weight.
- Greater tendency to pile on the pounds.

Why? In simple terms: when we sleep and when our body regenerates itself we produce two hormones: leptin and ghrelin. Since leptin curbs the appetite and ghrelin stimulates it and we produce more ghrelin and less leptin when we have less sleep, it is easy to understand how a lack of sleep can make us eat more by artificially increasing our appetite. Have you noticed that when you come back from a very late party, or after a sleepless night, you are extra hungry?

And if you think that catching up over the weekend is enough to compensate you are dead wrong. Studies are unanimous on this: two nights of too little sleep and the vicious circle is already in motion. In fact, a study conducted by the University of Chicago showed that after two days of sleep-deprivation, participants saw their leptin levels plummet, which, in turn, increased their appetite by a whopping 45 per cent! And, far from being attracted to apples, cucumbers or raw almonds, they were drawn to high-energy-dense foods like pizza, salty snacks, sweets, ice-cream and so on.

Don't become too zealous: sleeping more than your body needs won't curb your appetite, either. According to the most up-to-date consensus, you need seven to eight hours of quality sleep per night.

The solution: SLEEP MORE TO LOSE WEIGHT FASTER

In addition to your once-weekly screen fast, replace your daily soap opera with a book and turn off the lights before 11pm, and you'll very quickly observe an increase in your energy levels as well as a decrease in your stress levels (two days will suffice). Start tonight!

Consciously decide not to watch TV, or stay in front of your computer, or read emails after 7pm. Turn off all lights and block out all sources of noise before going to sleep. Don't watch TV or do work in bed. Learn how to wake up to your body's natural rhythm and not to an alarm clock, which can interrupt a phase of deep sleep. During the weekend (and during the week, if you work from home) give yourself the right to take an energising 30-minute nap (no more).

Checklist of SRAs
(Stress Reduction Actions)

1 Follow a strict news and social media fast on Sundays,
   or any other day of your choice.
2 List five energy vampires that prevent you from losing weight
   and eliminate them from your life (figuratively, of course!).
3 Practice abdominal breathing techniques (p. 42) when
   you wake up and before a majorly stressful event.
4 Give yourself a sleep makeover:

- Tonight, no TV. Choose a book right now, so you are prepared.
- Go to bed at 10pm, or when you feel tired – and not when
  the movie is over.
- Make sure that you sleep for seven to eight hours,
  six days per week.

ACTION PLAN AGAINST STRESS

I'm sure you have plenty more tips and ideas for beating stress,
that apply to your own personal situation. Write them down, below.
By doing this you will organise your thoughts around them and
they will become a part of your normal routine.

3   EXTERNAL POLLUTANTS

Lastly, let's talk about another source of toxins, which is pervasive and can't always be avoided: air pollution from cars, industry, chemical products and air-conditioning.

Unless you decide to retire to the virgin jungle it is very hard to escape ambient pollution. However, if you avoid exercising towards the end of the day, when the ozone and particle levels are at their peak, you will already be doing yourself more good in your quest for a toxin-free life. And if you are remodelling your house, make sure you use water-based paints and glues.

In warm weather, try to wean yourself off the air conditioning in your car by progressively increasing the temperature and getting used to not using it so much. In cold weather, do the opposite. This will help reduce the amount of moulds you inhale (because whatever the mechanic tells you, moulds form in any system that carries air and steam).

If you need to exercise when the pollution is at its peak, wear a scarf or handkerchief on your nose (as is normal practice in many Asian countries). You will be shocked to see how much soot there is on the fabric, after exercising!

Switch from standard household cleaning products (loaded with chemicals) to their natural, bio-degradable and environmentally-friendly counterparts.

25TH-HOUR EXERCISES

These exercises are designed to fit seamlessly into your hectic day by bringing the gym into your life, rather than the other way round. If you stand up regularly and squeeze these in, instead of staying seated at your desk for eight hours straight, you'll notice a huge difference in your fitness and body tone. They are also great for when you're detoxing heavily – if you've started with a very toxic body, you may be more tired than usual. Aim to fit in **five** every day.

Arm-wrestling
Here is an easy exercise to do at home if you have teenagers in the house or a partner who is game for it. Just ask them to challenge you to a special arm-wrestling game whereby your objective is not to win by touching down on the table, but rather to keep your arm in an upright position against theirs, without moving, for as long as you can. Aim to hold the position for 30 seconds, and then longer. Try to do this on a daily basis. You will be impressed by the feeling of force coursing through your veins and by how toned your biceps are after a few weeks.

Bathroom Squats
If you drink the right amount of water, Sobacha and tea each day, you will find that you need to go to the loo frequently, even if your bladder is very strong. Instead of sitting on the toilet seat, simply squat and stay in this position until you have 'finished'. If you do this quadriceps-strengthening exercise every time you go (at least six times a day), you will have the thighs of an Amazonian in a few weeks, I guarantee it!

The Brazilian
You can do this exercise while brushing your teeth! We spend, on average, six minutes a day cleaning our teeth – that's 42 minutes per week of buttock squeezes, the equivalent of a butt-firming class at the gym, without the sweat!

1   Stand up straight, feet hip-distance apart, and bend your knees slightly.
2   Keeping your abs tight and your back straight (no arching), tilt your hips forward while contracting your glutes. Make sure you give an extra hard squeeze as you do this!
3   Finish the move by pulling your hips back and releasing your glutes.
4   Repeat until the end of your brushing session.

Hindu Prayer

Breasts themselves aren't muscles so we can't tone them directly. We can, however, tone what I call the 'natural bra': our pectorals and an underlying muscle called the subscapularis, which is involved in lifting our breasts. I do this religiously (no pun intended) every single morning after my shower. Of course, you can decide to practise it at any point of the day   all you need is three minutes.

1   Stand in front of a mirror so that you can keep an eye on your posture, making sure you stay nice and straight.
2   Press your palms against each other, release and press again, moving them upwards as you do this.
3   Do a series of 20 presses above your head.
4   Slowly bring your hands down as you continue to press and release your palms against one another.
5   Repeat, moving up and down, until you reach 100 presses.

Iron Butt

Here is a move that allows you to isolate the buttock muscles so that you can work one after the other. You can do it at your desk very discreetly; nobody will notice anything!

1   Sit on a chair. Your left leg is in a normal pose with your foot flat on the ground. Your right leg is crossed over your left, with your right ankle resting on your left knee.
2   Contract the glute muscles on the right, crossed-leg side for 30 seconds. If you feel your right side trembling a little bit, go for 50 contractions on the same side, followed by 30 seconds of deep static contraction (this is what we call isometry).
3   Repeat on the other side.

Jumping Jacks

Do 50 of these every morning before eating breakfast, to boost your metabolism and burn calories. You can drink something first, but make sure you wait a short while before doing any jumping!

1 Stand with your legs together and arms straight down along your body.
2 As you jump, open your legs and bring your arms above your head so that your hands touch. You should land with your legs apart. Keep the knees flexed.
3 Finish the jump by returning to the starting position.

Open the Door to a Flat Tummy

Decide that each time you walk through a door, you'll suck in your abs. Once you associate the action and exercise, it'll become second nature – I contract my abs every time I walk through a doorway, without even thinking about it! Focus on contracting both your upper and lower abs (above and below your navel). You can also wear a red string or a band on your wrist that you associate with abdominal contractions, so that each time you look at it you'll be reminded to do some.

So, remember to contract your abs as often as possible, even when the phone rings, or while reading this book!

Permanent Contraction

This is my go-to for toning the buttocks. It's easy but (as always), highly efficient. Simply contract your glutes while you wait for the bus, between train station stops on your daily commute, at the red light, in work meetings (yes, it's discreet enough!) and while cooking, washing the car or folding laundry. You can truly do it any time, any place – even while you read this book! You can choose to contract 100 times quickly or slowly; or stay contracted for one minute straight; or contract one side first and then the other. It's up to you.

Walk while you Talk

Do you own a mobile phone (I bet the answer is yes!) or a cordless phone? How much time do you spend on the phone in a day? One hour? Two hours? More? I have calculated that I spend, on average, two hours on the phone every day – half of it sitting at my desk. I thus have one hour that I can use to walk about 6,000 steps. Put a Post-it on your phone that says, 'On the phone = walking'.

Just imagine how many steps you could take if you were constantly walking while talking on the phone!

If you work from home, then just walk around the block. At the office, walk around the building, in the hallways, or simply remain standing and switch from standing on one leg to standing on two. See how easy it is to squeeze in some activity? Make sure you have your pedometer on, so that you can see how many steps you have taken. Surprise yourself!

Whatever the case, always be on the move. You will burn more calories this way: three calories per minute for a slow-paced walk, two calories while standing, but only one calorie while sitting. A whole day of regular movement can actually amount to a hefty 500 calories burned, if not more (that's the equivalent of a small portion of fish and chips).

Wall Push-ups
Every time you go to the loo, take a moment to tone your triceps.

1   Stand in front of a wall, feet hip distance apart, close enough to touch it with your arms straight out, at eye level.

2   Place your palms on the wall and bend at the elbows to do 20 standing push-ups. Push your body back from the wall harder each time, moving slowly and maintaining control. Increase the difficulty of this exercise by keeping your fingers off the wall, or by working only one arm at a time.

TWO-WEEK DETOX DIET

Now that we have learned about the toxins we take in to our bodies through stress and external pollutants and those we generate as a result of an unbalanced diet, let's find out how we can eliminate them by means of our diet, with my two-week programme of intense detoxification. This will:

- Flush out toxins that make you feel sluggish.
- Increase your energy levels (essential for the phases that follow).
- Help you lose the first few pounds effortlessly and without depriving yourself.
- Give you back a glowing, peachy complexion.
- Establish a high level of motivation.

I ask that you follow the DETOX rules (page 27) as far as possible, as this phase is the cornerstone of my programme.

Just imagine you are preparing a used canvas for a new painting. Before painting over it and recreating the new you, you need to clear away the dust, remove the old paint and bleach the canvas (that's your DETOX phase) so that we have an amazing virgin canvas on which to draw up a healthy new life!

TWO WEEKS FOR EVERYBODY?

I am often asked why the DETOX phase lasts two weeks, no matter how many pounds you have to lose. Simply because, in the same way that you cannot make caramelised onions in 30 minutes (you need two whole hours for that!), you cannot cleanse your body faster than it takes to flush out the toxins. So, whether you have five or 50 pounds to lose, the same DETOX programme applies.

If your current diet is too light in fibre (fruit and vegetables), or if you are coming straight from a high-protein diet, it is very possible that these first two weeks will send you to the loo more often than usual. This is absolutely normal. It's also possible that the influx of fibre will give you a tummy ache. Add a bowl of white rice to each meal and then reduce that quantity until your bowel movements return to normal.

TOP 10 DETOX FOODS

1   Buckwheat

My miracle grain! You'll see that LeBootCamp Diet recommends a roasted buckwheat infusion called 'Sobacha' every morning, as it delivers so much goodness to the body. Despite its name, buckwheat bears absolutely no relation to wheat. It belongs to the same family as rhubarb and sorrel and can be traced back to Siberia, Northern China and Japan. Buckwheat was brought to Europe during the Middle Ages by the Crusaders, who had seen 'Saracens' (as they called Middle-Eastern people) using it – hence its French name, 'sarraoin'. This plant is naturally organic because growing it requires no fungicides, herbicides or pesticides – another reason why I love it. It is good for the body and good for the planet! Check out '10 Reasons to Love Buckwheat' (p. 55).

2   Apple

Like buckwheat, the apple is a very affordable detox food. Go for seasonal organic apples to avoid those very pesticides and chemical products that we are trying to rid our body of! Apples are an excellent source of vitamin C. They also contain quercetin (a flavonoid and one of the numerous pigment molecules that gives colour to fruits, vegetables and medicinal plants) and pectin, a fibre which binds itself to heavy metals like mercury or lead in the colon and supports their excretion. Pectin also helps our body excrete preservatives and other food additives, including tartrazine, which has been linked to hyperactivity, migraines and asthma. Finally, pectin is a water-soluble fibre which swells in our stomach when it comes into contact with liquids, thereby inducing a feeling of fullness. For this reason I recommend eating an apple 20 minutes in advance of a meal at a restaurant or a buffet!

FACT An apple a day keeps the doctor away! The apple is so detoxifying that Russian doctors made irradiated children from Chernobyl eat apples. Indeed, many researchers, including Professor V.B. Nesterenko, of the Institute for Radioprotection 'Belrad' in Belarus, established that the pectin contained in apples can help reduce radiation levels in children's bodies.

3   Artichoke

Artichoke increases the production of bile. Since one of the missions of bile is to transport toxins to the intestinal tract where they will be excreted, the more bile, the better.

Recent studies have shown that 30 minutes after the consumption of one artichoke, the production of bile increased by a whopping 100 per cent. Not bad, hey?

A word of caution: never keep a cooked artichoke to eat later on. Just like broccoli or spinach, this vegetable actually releases toxins when exposed to air and light, and can thus even become toxic. How ironic when you are going through a detox phase!

> NOTE Conventional guidelines recommend that cooked artichokes and broccoli can be kept for up to three days. Nutrition experts – such as myself – would suggest keeping them for no longer than 12 hours.

4   Avocado

I love avocados because they are rich in healthy fats, so half an avocado (without added mayonnaise, of course) will do you good. If you add prawns and a little bit of soy sauce, you will have a tasty and well-balanced dish. Avocado contains glutathione: if you haven't yet heard of this, it is because the studies on this antioxidant are still very few. Glutathione enables the transformation of fat-stored toxins into water-soluble toxins, making them easy to eliminate. Also, according to a recent study conducted by Harvard Medical School, over-60s who consumed a lot of avocado (i.e., one a day) suffered less from arthrosis than people who did not consume avocado (with all else being equal).

5   Banana

A staple food, and very inexpensive. Always choose organic because the cultivation of conventional bananas is simply an ecological calamity (along with apples, bananas are one of the crops most heavily treated with chemicals). It's also a medical disaster for those living on the plantations because they are, literally, walking in pesticide-loaded mud. Thanks to the purchasing power of supermarkets, bananas remain very affordable, even when organic. Bananas are a fantastic source of potassium, which helps regulate the fluids levels in our body. The equation is very simple: the more fluids retained in our body, the more toxins are stored; so, the fewer fluids, the fewer toxins.

6 Beetroot

Once again, a detox food that's totally affordable and easy to find!
I prefer raw beetroots to cooked ones, but this is just a question of
taste as they both provide amazing antioxidants such as methionine
and betanin. Methionine helps the body purify itself of toxic waste
and betanin helps the liver metabolise fatty acids, thus allowing our
liver to concentrate on more dangerous toxins.

7 Cruciferae

The cruciferae family includes cabbage, Brussels sprouts, spinach,
watercress, cauliflower, kale, pak choi, and other lesser-known
vegetables such as romanesco broccoli, which I particularly love.
Easy to find and easy to cook, cruciferous vegetables are a great gift
of nature. Whether you eat them raw or not, their potent compounds
neutralise nitrosamines (toxic agents produced by cigarette smoke).
So, for each cigarette puff, one spinach salad!

Brussels sprouts also inhibit aflatoxin, a very toxic mould that has
been linked to liver cancer.

With its light, peppery taste and its rich antioxidant content,
watercress is a marvel of nature. It contains chlorophyll, which
supports the production of red blood cells. A recent study has
shown that smokers who consumed watercress daily (one salad
a day) excreted more toxins in their urine than smokers who did
not eat watercress (but iceberg lettuce, instead).

8 Garlic

Garlic is a detox powerhouse and should be crushed to activate potent,
beneficial enzymes such as allicin. This organosulfur helps our body
maintain its pH balance (pp. 181–195) and can help fight cravings in
smokers who are trying to quit. It binds itself to toxins like mercury
and food additives and helps the body excrete them. So, don't hesitate
to add crushed garlic to your salads and home-cooked meals. You can
also cut a garlic head in half and roast it in the oven at 190°C/375°F/
gas mark 5 for around 20 minutes – divine!

9 Prunes

Ideal for satisfying sweet cravings, prunes contain three powerful
active ingredients that work together in an amazing manner: tartaric
acid and diphenyl isatin, both natural laxatives, and a type of alcohol
sugar called sorbitol that can loosen the stool. Easier and more

frequent bowel movements support your body's natural detoxifying functions. Plus, prunes contain a high level of vitamin C, which supports iron absorption – good news for women who are chronically iron deficient (anaemic).

NOTE Eat prunes in moderation, as they contain high levels of sugar.

10 Tofu

While tofu was never a classic staple in Europe, its popularity is steadily growing. Tofu is an amazing protein source without any saturated fat. You can replace red meat with tofu in a vegetarian chilli, or you can sauté it with onions and garlic, soy sauce and brown rice for an Asian dish.

Although studies on tofu's detoxifying properties are limited, they reveal that tofu binds itself to heavy metals and helps the body eliminate them. A Harvard Medical School study showed that people who consumed tofu daily (I know, that seems like a lot!) had 10 per cent fewer toxins in their body.

NOTE There has been some debate over whether the risk of breast cancer can be increased by soy products like tofu; but this is a controversial and evolving area, and the latest research showed no conclusive evidence to support this.

KEEPING TRACK OF YOUR WEIGHT

Weigh yourself on the first day of your two-week DETOX and then at least every other day, in the morning on an empty stomach and after your first bowel movement of the day. Record your weight on 'Your weight-loss progress page' at the end of this book (page 244). Do not worry if your weight loss is not linear and constant. The body is NOT a machine and your efforts might take a few days to show results on the scale. To evaluate your progress better I suggest that, in addition to weighing yourself, you measure your body fat (scales offering this function are becoming more and more affordable), as well as your thighs, waist and arm circumference.

10 REASONS TO LOVE BUCKWHEAT

1 It's easy to cook, with a delicious, nutty taste.

2 For its high protein content: buckwheat contains all the essential amino acids – a rarity in nature. Combined with a source of vegetable protein like pulses, it can completely replace any source of animal protein.

3 Unlike wheat or even some types of oats, it contains no gluten, so it's recommended for people suffering from coeliac disease and gluten-sensitive individuals (like me!).

4 For its high fibre content, which helps you feel fuller faster and reduces cholesterol and blood sugar levels.

5 For its low glycaemic index – lower, in fact, than almost all cereal products. And we know that a low glycaemic index helps reduce storage of sugar in the form of fat (pp. 98–103).

6 Because it contains vitamins P, B1, B3, B5, B6, all of which are excellent for our hair and skin health. These vitamins also help fight against symptoms caused by excess stress, as well as support our immune system and increase our metabolism.

7 For its wealth of trace elements: buckwheat contains more fluor, copper, magnesium, manganese, phosphorus, zinc and iron than wheat.

8 Because a study comparing the composition of buckwheat to that of wheat, oats, rye and barley, shows that buckwheat has a higher antioxidant content than any other grain.

9 Because buckwheat contains several phenolic acids, which are potent antioxidants not affected by heat and transformation (i.e., cutting, puréeing, blending). Phenolic acids can help protect against certain cancers and cardiovascular diseases.

10 For its high content of flavonoids (powerful antioxidants). Rutin, for example, has anti-inflammatory properties and can help strengthen blood vessels.

DETOX
FOOD GUIDE

Foods to avoid

- Cow dairy
- Eggs and mayonnaise
- Red meat
- Gluten
- Yeast
- Alcohol
- Carnivorous and predatory fish (even wild fish, because of mercury)
- Non-organic fruits and vegetables
- Rich sauces and heavy foods
- Sugar products
- All foods containing high-fructose corn syrup
- Aspartame and other potentially unsafe chemical sweeteners (pp. 33–37)
- Fizzy drinks (whether regular or diet)
- Processed food products containing additives that may be harmful
- Processed biscuits, cakes, sweets and ready meals

Foods to enjoy

- Sheep and goat dairy
- White meat
- Small fish (wild or organically farmed), like anchovies and sardines
- Wild, large fish from protected areas like Alaska
- Seafood
- Organic potato and sweet potato
- Buckwheat, whole cereals and grains
- Pulses
- Organic soy
- Vegan yogurts (made from almond, coconut, rice and hemp milks)
- Mustard
- Nuts
- Olive oil in small quantities
- Prunes and other dried fruits (organic and without sulphur dioxide)
- Seeds
- Homemade, organic fruit juices
- Dark chocolate (70 per cent cocoa solids)
- Agave syrup
- Honey
- Stevia and erythritol (natural, low-calorie sweeteners)

Foods to feast on

- Organic fruits, especially apples, bananas, berries, citruses, peaches
- Organic vegetables, especially artichokes, asparagus, avocados, beetroot, cruciferous veg, garlic, green beans, mushrooms, peas, tomatoes
- Organic roots, especially carrots, Jerusalem artichokes, swede, turnips
- Sobacha (roasted, infused buckwheat; p. 71)
- Green, white and herbal teas
- All spices (make sure they are not UV-treated)
- All herbs (same caution as for spices)
- Low-sugar, low-salt pickled vegetables (cabbage, carrots, cauliflower, cucumber)
- Seaweeds
- Sprouted seeds
- Tofu

DETOX MENUS

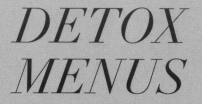

I have created these menus with all the DETOX principles in mind: using detoxifying foods from my top 10 list (plus some other foods which have detox properties but did not make it to the top 10); avoiding gluten and red meat – but still delivering plenty of flavour. Some of my recipes can be eaten across the phases, so there are a couple of menu suggestions from other chapters.

There's no wine allowed in DETOX, but don't worry – once you've reached the ATTACK phase, you can enjoy a daily glass of red!

The menus are suggestions only. If you cannot follow them because you are allergic to some ingredients, or because you work long hours in an office, just pick the options which work for you. If you prefer to eat one of the dinners for lunch, this is completely fine. Repeating meals that you particularly like is also acceptable.

The tips, below, will not only help you get the most out of your two-week DETOX phase, but are also important principles for every phase in this book. By MAINTENANCE, they will be part of your life.

Bon appétit!

Healthy cooking methods

The healthiest way is always to enjoy fruits and veggies raw (not counting the tomato, which develops antioxidants as it is cooked). After this, cooking methods should be in this order of preference: steam briefly, grill or bake, boil. Boiling comes last because we lose the vast majority of nutrients in the water we discard. The worst way to cook remains the microwave – after two minutes (on high) it destroys more than 98 per cent of vitamins!

Choose organic

Remember to choose organic fish, meat, fruit and veg, where possible.

Season sparingly

Always use sea salt – Fleur de Sel or Maldon salt, for preference. Use it sparingly, and add fresh herbs whenever you like, for flavour.

Remember portion size

While the amount of fruits and vegetables you can eat are unlimited, one portion of fish or meat should never exceed 100–120g per meal. If you have a hard time determining this without weighing, try equating the portion size to a full pack of 52 cards:

- One portion of meat or fish is equivalent to one pack
- One portion of cheese is half a pack
- One portion of sweets, biscuits and other rich foods is half a pack

If you don't have a playing card deck within reach, you can also use the palm of your hand, which is approximately the same size.

Feast, not famine

I'm completely against deprivation in LeBootCamp Diet. Sure, there are foods that we need to limit in all phases – particularly in DETOX and BOOSTER; but being too strict is counter-productive, as it leads to frustration and can undermine your motivation. This is why I have introduced the concept of **Feast.** You'll see this wherever there are fresh fruit and veg, which you can enjoy freely, or a super-healthy recipe where you really don't need to be strict about portion size (just remember not to increase oil or margarine quantities, if the recipe calls for them). There is always room for the occasional uplifting treat, so I've included chocolate as a snack on a few days. This will make you happy, meaning you'll produce fewer toxins! Have dark if you prefer, but milk chocolate is fine, too.

Dairy and calcium

You will notice that my menus feature hardly any dairy products. This is because, during DETOX, we try and avoid all cow dairy. You are, no doubt, wondering where you will get your calcium from? Despite what TV ads tell us about dairy products being an indispensable source of calcium, they are, in fact, not the only source, nor even the best one! Otherwise, how would the Japanese, who consume very little, or no dairy, survive? What's more, statistically, they have three times fewer bone fractures than the rest of the world. Remember that we are the only mammals that consume the milk from other mammals for the sake of strong bones. This has not always been the case, so how did our ancestors manage?

Suffice to say, that we can get all the calcium we need from other foods, such as dark leafy greens, sesame seeds, anchovies, salmon, dry figs and some mineral waters.

DAY 1

BREAKFAST

Juice of ½ lemon in 125ml
room-temperature water
1 cup Sobacha (p. 71)
1 Buckwheat Crêpe (p. 71)
1 tbsp strawberry jam
1 vegan yoghurt (coconut, rice or soya milk)
Feast: pink grapefruit (see p. 88), or orange

LUNCH

1 grilled salmon fillet with shallot (sauté
chopped shallot in olive oil, remove from pan,
sauté salmon, then return shallot to pan)
1 steamed potato mashed with 1 tbsp
olive oil
1 Blue Boost (p. 72)

SNACK

10 raw almonds
Feast: apple

DINNER

Tomato Soup with Edamame (p. 78)
Stir-fried Tofu with Dijon Mustard (p. 80)
1 slice toasted gluten-free, yeast-free bread
1 orange

DAY 2

BREAKFAST

Juice of ½ lemon in 125ml
room-temperature water
1 cup Sobacha (p. 71)
1 Buckwheat Crêpe (p. 71)
1 tbsp prune jam
1 smoothie made with Hazelnut Milk (p. 73),
1 banana and seasonal berries

LUNCH

Chicken breast grilled with lemon juice,
curry powder and fresh coriander
Feast: pumpkin or squash, diced and
baked with 1 tbsp olive oil
Feast: oranges

SNACK

10 raw almonds
Feast: pears

DINNER

Steamed artichoke with Yogurt Sauce (p. 80)
Feast: Brussels Sprouts with Green Tea (p. 77)
Grilled fish with 1 tbsp olive oil and Provençal
herbs (or fresh herbs of your choice)
5 prunes

DAY 3

BREAKFAST

Juice of ½ lemon in 125ml
room-temperature water
1 cup Sobacha (p. 71)
1 Buckwheat Crêpe (p. 71)
1 tbsp strawberry jam
1 banana
Feast: pink grapefruit (see p. 88), or orange

LUNCH

Salad of watercress with shredded red
cabbage and Garlic Vinaigrette (p. 82)
1 small tin wild tuna with fresh basil and
balsamic vinegar
5 tbsp steamed quinoa with marinara sauce
(cooked, peeled tomatoes; drizzle of olive oil;
salt, pepper and basil)
1 vegan yogurt (coconut, rice or soy milk)

SNACK

10 hazelnuts or almonds
4 squares chocolate (your favourite)
2 kiwis

DINNER

1 veal escalope brushed with wholegrain
mustard and grilled
Mashed, steamed broccoli with 1 tbsp
olive oil
Feast: fresh, seasonal fruit salad

DAY 4

BREAKFAST

Juice of ½ lemon in 125ml
room-temperature water
1 cup Sobacha (p. 71)
Small bowl muesli, plus 1 vegan yoghurt
(coconut, rice or soy milk)
Feast: cubed apple with cinnamon

LUNCH

Grilled red mullet
Feast: salad of mushrooms marinated
in lemon and basil
1 slice gluten-free, yeast-free bread
1 banana

SNACK

1 Buckwheat Crêpe (p. 71)
Feast: seasonal berries

DINNER

4 tbsp Hummus (p. 76)
1 corn tortilla
1 steamed artichoke with Soyannaise (p. 81)
Feast: Grapefruit-strawberry Mix (p. 88)

DAY 5

BREAKFAST

Juice of ½ lemon in 125ml
room temperature water
1 cup Sobacha (p. 71)
1 Buckwheat Crêpe (p. 71)
1 tbsp strawberry jam
1 orange plus 10 raw almonds

LUNCH

Grilled-veggie sandwich on gluten-free,
yeast-free bread, with 1 tbsp olive oil
2 slices cooked turkey
1 banana

SNACK

1 corn tortilla
2 tbsp Hummus (p. 76)
5 prunes

DINNER

Feast: salad of watercress with
Garlic Vinaigrette (p. 82)
Grilled salmon fillet with lemon
1 slice gluten-free, yeast-free toast
4 squares chocolate (your favourite)

DAY 6

BREAKFAST

Juice of ½ lemon in 125ml
room-temperature water
1 cup Sobacha (p. 71)
1 Buckwheat Crêpe (p. 71) with 3 tbsp
homemade apple purée (peeled, chopped
apples cooked gently with a splash of water)
Feast: pink grapefruit (see p. 88), or orange

LUNCH

½ avocado with Soyannaise (p. 81)
1 small portion Carrot Salad with
Raisins (p. 78)
2 grilled, fresh sardines
1 slice gluten-free, yeast-free toast
4 squares chocolate (your favourite)

SNACK

1 Buckwheat Crêpe (p. 71)
10 raw almonds

DINNER

Feast: Rocket and Broccoli Soup (p. 75)
4 tbsp steamed quinoa
2 slices ham or turkey ham
Feast: seasonal fresh fruit salad

DAY 7

BREAKFAST

Juice of ½ lemon in 125ml
room-temperature water
1 cup Sobacha (p. 71)
1 Buckwheat Crêpe (p. 71) with 3 tbsp
apple purée (homemade, as for Day 6)
Fruit salad of prunes and kiwi

LUNCH

Smoked Salmon Rolls with Cream Cheese
(p. 84)
Feast: Courgette and Caramelised
Onion Gratin (p. 77)
1 banana

SNACK

4 tbsp vegan or lactose-free cottage cheese
with 1 tbsp raw, organic honey

DINNER

Feast: sautéed tofu with Tomato Coulis (p. 227)
5 tbsp steamed brown rice
Feast: carrot and split pea purée (with 1 tbsp
non-hydrogenated margarine, salt and
pinch nutmeg)
1 pear

DAY 8

BREAKFAST

Juice of ½ lemon in 125ml
room-temperature water
1 cup Sobacha (p. 71)
1 Buckwheat Crêpe (p. 71)
1 banana, sliced, with coconut flakes

LUNCH

Grilled or steamed white fish with
steamed carrots
Steamed Brussels sprouts with 1 tbsp
olive oil
Feast: Tri-colour Fruit Salad (p. 89)

SNACK

1 Buckwheat Crêpe (p. 71)
3 dried figs

DINNER

Chicken with Lemon and Cumin (p. 85)
with 3 tbsp steamed brown rice
Feast: salad of watercress with Garlic
Vinaigrette (p. 82)
Feast: clementines or satsumas
Note: soak almonds in water overnight,
ready for snack on Day 9

DAY 9

BREAKFAST

Juice of ½ lemon in 125ml
room-temperature water
1 cup Sobacha (p. 71)
1 Buckwheat Crêpe (p. 71)
Purple Milkshake (p. 74)

LUNCH

Feast: salad of shredded green cabbage
with Lemon Vinaigrette (p. 83)
2 slices white turkey meat
1 slice gluten-free, yeast-free bread
1 banana

SNACK

1 apple plus 10 raw, sprouted almonds
(see Dinner, Day 8)
4 dried figs

DINNER

Feta and Olive Pasta Salad (p. 87)
Feast: salad of sliced, cooked beetroot
with Lemon Vinaigrette (p. 83)
Feast: pink grapefruit (see p. 88), or orange

DAY 10

BREAKFAST

Juice of ½ lemon in 125ml
room-temperature water
1 cup Sobacha (p. 71)
1 Buckwheat Crêpe (p. 71)
1 tbsp strawberry jam
1 Green Morning Boost (p. 73)

LUNCH

Feast: pink grapefruit (see p. 88), or orange
Feast: salad of baby spinach, shredded
red cabbage, apple and artichoke hearts
with Garlic Vinaigrette (p. 82)
1 piece white chicken meat
1 slice gluten-free, yeast-free bread

SNACK

1 Buckwheat Crêpe (p. 71)
1 banana

DINNER

Feast: cooked beetroot, watercress,
½ avocado and Garlic Vinaigrette (p. 82)
1 steamed potato mashed with 1 tbsp olive oil
1 grilled Vegetarian Burger (p. 237)
4 squares chocolate (your favourite)

DAY 11

BREAKFAST

Juice of ½ lemon in 125ml
room-temperature water
1 cup Sobacha (p. 71)
1 Date Smoothie (p. 72)

LUNCH

Avocado and Salmon Tortilla (p. 84)
Feast: rocket and watercress salad
with Lemon Vinaigrette (p. 83)
1 pear

SNACK

1 Buckwheat Crêpe (p. 71)
10 raw hazelnuts

DINNER

Ratatouille Provençale (p. 79)
2 slices white turkey meat
1 slice gluten-free, yeast-free bread
Feast: apple, raisin and walnut salad with
Balsamic Vinaigrette (p. 82)

DAY 12

BREAKFAST

Juice of ½ lemon in 125ml
room-temperature water
1 cup Sobacha (p. 71)
1 Buckwheat Crêpe (p. 71) with 3 tbsp
apple purée (homemade, as for Day 6)
1 soy yogurt
a few grapes

LUNCH

Steamed fish (your choice)
Feast: garlic-carrot purée (for 4, blend
500g cooked carrots with 2 tbsp
non-hydrogenated margarine, seasoning,
crushed garlic clove and pinch of nutmeg)
1 slice gluten-free, yeast-free bread
a few lychees

SNACK

1 banana smoothie (250ml non-dairy milk,
1 banana, 1 tsp vanilla extract, 1 tbsp
agave nectar)
10 raw hazelnuts

DINNER

1 leg Chicken Tandoori (p. 86)
Feast: green peas
3 tbsp Raita (p. 80)
½ gluten-free, yeast-free pitta or naan bread
1 satsuma or clementine

DAY 13

BREAKFAST

Juice of ½ lemon in 125ml room-temperature water

1 cup Sobacha (p. 71)

1 Buckwheat Crêpe (p. 71) with 3 tbsp apple purée

1 tbsp raw, organic honey with a knife-end of butter

Feast: Grapefruit-strawberry Mix (p. 88) (or any seasonal fruits)

LUNCH

Trout Fillet in Hazelnut Crust (p. 85)

Feast: salad of watercress and lamb's lettuce with vinaigrette of your choice (pp. 82–83)

1 slice gluten-free, yeast-free bread

1 plain, vegan yogurt

SNACK

10 raw walnuts

1 banana

3 dried figs

DINNER

Tuna tartine (1 slice gluten-free, yeast-free toast topped with tuna, 1 tbsp Soyannaise and 1 tsp vinegar)

Beetroot and sweetcorn salad (to be eaten AFTER the tuna tartine)

Small bowl fruit purée of your choice

DAY 14

BREAKFAST

Juice of ½ lemon in 125ml
room-temperature water
1 cup Sobacha (p. 71)
1 Buckwheat Crêpe (p. 71) with 3 tbsp
apple purée (homemade, as for Day 6)
1 Kiwi, Grape and Asian Pear Boost (p. 74)

LUNCH

Carrot Salad with Raisins (p. 78), with a
few cubes of ham
½ avocado with Soyannaise (p. 81)
1 slice rye bread
3 tbsp apple purée

SNACK

1 Buckwheat Crêpe (p. 71)
1 plain, vegan yogurt with 1 tbsp raw,
organic honey

DINNER

Feast: Spinach, Strawberry and Apple Salad
(p. 88)
Vegetarian Burger (p. 207) with 5 tbsp
steamed quinoa
Feast: blueberries or other seasonal berries

DETOX
RECIPES

SOBACHA

Serves 1
Preparation 5 min

Ingredients
2 tbsp kasha
(roasted buckwheat
seeds)
250ml boiled water

This infusion (also known as soba-cha) is made from roasted buckwheat, and is widely drunk in Japan. Of all the grains, buckwheat is the richest in magnesium. Magnesium strengthens the body's capacity to resist stress, but studies show that most people don't consume enough. Here's the solution: a small cup of buckwheat infusion every day and you will feel relaxed and ready to face any stressful situation!

If you can only find raw buckwheat seeds, roast them in a dry frying pan over medium heat, until golden. If you're really pressed for time, try a Sobacha tisane – such as the one I've designed for when I'm at work or travelling (see www.VOlifestyle.co.uk).

1   Put the buckwheat seeds in a small teapot or cup. Add the water and leave to infuse for 5 minutes.

2   Strain into another cup before drinking.

BUCKWHEAT CRÊPES

Serves 2
Preparation 5 min

Ingredients
40g buckwheat flour
120ml water
pinch of salt
canola oil, for
greasing, if
necessary

This easy, gluten-free recipe is a key component of LeBootCamp Diet. You can make the batter the night before and keep it, covered, in the fridge. Serve with organic, raw honey; a tiny spoonful of low-GI strawberry jam or non-hydrogenated margarine. Add a piece of fruit and you've a healthy breakfast rich in prebiotics that will help you lose weight and keep you going until lunch. (See p. 225 for a non-buckwheat version).

1   Place all the ingredients in a large bowl.

2   Whisk until you have a smooth batter.

3   Heat a small, non-stick or lightly oiled frying pan and add half the mixture, using a ladle. Tip to spread across the surface.

4   Cook for 2-3 minutes. Turn the crêpe and cook the other side.

5   Set aside and keep warm while you make the second crêpe.

BLUE BOOST

Serves 1
Preparation 5 min

Ingredients
1 cup blueberries
(wild is best)
5 strawberries
1 apple
½ cup blackberries
(if you can't get
blackberries,
replace with more
blueberries)

Containing strawberries, blackberries and blueberries, the Blue Boost brings you plenty of much-needed nutrients and phytochemicals. I haven't given exact measures here, as it really doesn't matter if they aren't precise: just use a large tea cup or mug. If you don't have a juicer, I strongly advise you buy one! You can use a blender, then strain the juice through a very fine sieve, but it won't taste so good.

1   Rinse and pat dry all fruits.

2   Put the fruits directly into the juicer – no need to peel.

3   Juice and drink right away as antioxidants lose their potency as time passes.

DATE SMOOTHIE

Serves 1
Preparation 5 min

Ingredients
1 glass vegan milk
(hemp, rice, almond
or soy)
4 dates, pitted
1 tbsp agave nectar
(or 1 packet of
splenda)
½ tsp vanilla extract
½ avocado

Instead of reaching for that cake or dessert, try this smoothie – it's a delicious and healthy way to satisfy sugar cravings. Dates are certainly rich but there are only four in this, so it won't make the scale tip in the wrong direction. Dates are an amazing source of potassium and fibre, while avocados are packed with much-needed vitamin E and help keep our skin supple and healthy.

1   Place all the ingredients in your blender and pulse until fully puréed.

2   Pour into a large glass and enjoy!

GREEN MORNING BOOST

Serves 1
Preparation 5 min

Ingredients
1 apple
2 carrots
½ cucumber
1 stalk celery
1 handful kale
2 slices fresh ginger

I call this a 'green' boost because the majority of the ingredients are green. However, when everything has been juiced, the colour of the carrots dominates, and it ends up being more of a mix between green and orange.

1　Rinse the apple and vegetables and pat dry.

2　Put everything directly into the juicer – no need to peel.

3　Juice and drink right away.

HAZELNUT MILK

Serves 1
Preparation 5 min, plus overnight soaking

Ingredients
1 handful of fresh hazelnuts, soaked in water overnight
½ tsp vanilla extract (or less, if you prefer a subtler vanilla taste)
1 tbsp agave nectar or raw, organic honey; or splenda or stevia (optional)

Here is a way to enjoy 'milk', without any of the concerns related to dairy products, such as lactose-intolerance. Easily digested and original, hazelnut milk is easy to make and is a fantastic source of enzymes good for your health. My son, who is a good test, adores it!

1　The night before, soak the hazelnuts in a bowl of water. Make sure they are completely covered in water as they will expand slightly overnight.

2　In the morning, rinse and drain the hazelnuts. Put them in a blender with 2-3 times their volume of water and blend until you have a milky-white liquid.

3　Filter the milk through very fine filter paper, or a nut milk bag, to eliminate pulp.

4　Add the vanilla extract. Stir in the agave nectar or honey, or other sweeteners.

KIWI, GRAPE AND ASIAN PEAR BOOST

Serves 1
Preparation 5 min

Ingredients
1 Asian pear, unpeeled
12 grapes
½ cucumber, unpeeled
1 kiwi, peeled

You will need a juicer for this boost. I prefer to use Asian pears, as they are really juicy. However, you could use 2–3 conference pears instead if you can't find them.

1   Rinse the pear, grapes and cucumber and dry them. Cut the pear in half (or in quarters, if the mouth of your juicer is on the small side), and core.

2   Run all the ingredients through the juicer and enjoy right away.

PURPLE MILKSHAKE

Serves 2
Preparation 2 min

Ingredients
450g fresh or slightly thawed blueberries
115g soy yogurt
½ tsp stevia, or to taste
3 drops vanilla extract
250ml soy milk (or any other vegan milk)
8 ice cubes

This tasty little pleasure is sweet, easy and quick to prepare. It contains a nice amount of muscle-building protein and antioxidants. Researchers have found that blueberries rank top in terms of antioxidant activity when compared with 40 other fresh fruits and vegetables. As we know, antioxidants help neutralise 'free radicals' – by-products of metabolism that can lead to cancer and other age-related diseases. Anthocyanin – the pigment that makes blueberries blue – is thought to be responsible for this major health benefit. This makes a wonderful drink for children (and is a healthy alternative to processed juices).

1   Put all the ingredients in the blender.

2   Blend and drink.

Serving suggestion: serve with an avocado sandwich for a well-balanced meal that's low in saturated fat.

ROCKET AND
BROCCOLI SOUP

Serves 2
Preparation 15 min

Ingredients
1 head broccoli
1 small packet
rocket
1 tbsp olive oil
salt and freshly
ground pepper,
to taste
goat's cheese or
coconut cream, to
serve (optional)

A special thank you to my London friend, Selina, who shared this tasty recipe with me. For a main course, serve this soup with prawns or smoked salmon.

1   Bring a pan of water to the boil and add a pinch of salt.

2   Wash the broccoli and chop into even pieces, then add to the water. Add the rocket. The water should just cover the broccoli and rocket.

3   As soon as the broccoli is soft (after about 5 minutes; you want it to be bright green still) remove the pan from the hob.

4   Carefully pour the contents of the pan into the food processor and purée until smooth. You might want to reserve some of the water if you like your soup quite thick, like I do – you can always add it later to adjust the consistency.

5   Add a drizzle of olive oil, plus salt and pepper, to taste.

6   Serve each bowl of soup with 1 tsp fresh goat's cheese or coconut cream, if you wish.

Variation: you can replace the water with organic vegetable stock.

TOMATO SOUP WITH EDAMAME

Serves 1
Preparation 5 min

Ingredients
475ml tomato soup
(preferably fresh
and organic, but
from a tin will work
as well)
20 frozen or fresh
edamame beans
(soybeans), shelled
fresh oregano or
basil, to garnish

Make this colourful soup in a snap. It provides healthy fibre and the highest level of cancer-fighting lycopene. Choose a soup that is not loaded with sugar or, better still, contains no sugar at all. If it contains salt then make sure you don't add any at the end. If you don't have edamame, broad beans will work fine, as will peas.

1   Heat the tomato soup until serving temperature is reached.

2   Warm up the edamame beans in a pan with a tiny amount of water.

3   Pour the soup into a serving bowl.

4   Sprinkle edamame beans and oregano or basil over the soup.

HUMMUS

Serves 2
Preparation 5 min

Ingredients
1 x 400g tin organic,
cooked chickpeas
juice of ½ lemon
75ml extra-virgin
olive oil, plus more
½ tsp tahini paste
(sesame paste)
1 garlic clove
2 tsp cumin
salt, to taste
olives and flat-leaf
parsley, to garnish
(optional)

This tasty and very healthy dip is one that I recommend you always keep ready in your fridge to satisfy your salty/fibre cravings. It can also be used as a spread or served as a side dish.

1   Put all the ingredients in a blender, apart from the olives and parsley. Blend until you have a coarse or smooth purée, as you prefer.

2   To serve, put the mixture in a serving bowl. Pour some olive oil on top and garnish with a few olives and parsley, if you wish.

Variations:
•   Add 5 sun-dried tomatoes
•   Leave out the tahini (sesame paste)
•   Add 100g fresh, white mushrooms

Be creative!

BRUSSELS SPROUTS WITH GREEN TEA

This is a great detox recipe from the ever-popular cruciferous family. Delicious with grilled chicken or turkey.

Serves 2
Preparation 30 min

Ingredients
500g Brussels sprouts, rinsed
1 ½ tbsp non-hydrogenated margarine
2 small onions, sliced
500ml green tea
salt and freshly ground black pepper
½ tsp cinnamon
½ tsp ground cloves
1 spring onion, finely chopped

1   Cut each Brussels sprouts into quarters.

2   In a frying pan, heat the margarine and sear the onions until golden brown. Add the Brussels sprouts.

3   When the Brussels sprouts start caramelising and there is no juice left in the pan, add 125ml green tea, scraping the bottom of the pan.

4   Season with salt, pepper, the spices and spring onion.

5   Gradually add more tea and keep adding until the Brussels sprouts are fully cooked.

COURGETTE AND CARAMELISED ONION GRATIN

Serves 2
Preparation 1 hour 20 min

Ingredients
2 tbsp olive oil
1 onion, sliced
pinch of sugar or ½ tsp raw, organic honey
½ garlic clove, crushed
1 courgette, sliced but not peeled
2 medium tomatoes, sliced
1 bay leaf
thyme, salt and pepper, to taste

1   Heat 1 tbsp oil in a large pan over low heat and cook the onion until caramelised. This should take around 45 minutes, so you could use the time to contract your glutes or abs! When the onion starts turning brown, add the sugar or honey.

2   Preheat the oven to 180°C/350°F/gas mark 4.

3   Sprinkle an oiled dish with the garlic.

4   Layer the courgette and tomato slices, alternating to form a pattern.

5   Add the bay leaf and top with the caramelised onions.

6   Sprinkle over some thyme, salt and pepper and drizzle with the remaining 1 tbsp olive oil.

7   Bake for 30 minutes. Serve hot.

STIR-FRIED TOFU WITH DIJON MUSTARD

This delicious vegetarian dish is my son's favourite. Serve with wild or brown rice and a watercress salad.

Serves 1
Preparation 15 min, plus marinading time

Ingredients
110g firm tofu
1 tsp Dijon mustard
2 tbsp balsamic vinegar
2 tbsp soy sauce
2 tbsp olive oil
1 garlic clove, crushed
salt and freshly ground black pepper

1　Cube the tofu and put in a bowl. Coat in the mustard, balsamic vinegar, soy sauce and olive oil. Add crushed garlic, salt and pepper.

2　Cover and place in the fridge to marinate all day, or for at least 4 hours.

3　Sauté over high heat in a non-stick frying pan for 10 minutes (there's no need to add any extra oil but you can add a little of the marinade to the pan, as necessary, to prevent the tofu cubes from burning).

CARROT SALAD WITH RAISINS

Serves 1
Preparation 10 min

Ingredients
1 large carrot
1 handful raisins
1 tsp Soyannaise (p. 81)
1 tsp balsamic vinegar
1 tsp canola oil
salt and freshly ground black pepper
fresh parsley, to garnish

1　Peel and grate the carrot and put into a large salad bowl.

2　Add the raisins and mix.

3　Prepare a vinaigrette with the Soyannaise, vinegar, oil and seasoning.

4　Add the vinaigrette to salad and mix.

5　Garnish with the parsley and serve immediately so that the carrots do not become soggy.

RATATOUILLE PROVENÇALE

Serves 4
Preparation 1 hour
30 min

Ingredients
750g tomatoes
500g courgettes
2 medium
aubergines
½ green pepper
½ red pepper
½ yellow pepper
1½ onions
3 garlic cloves
3 sage leaves,
finely chopped
(or 1 tsp dried)
fresh basil, finely
chopped, to taste
2-3 tbsp olive oil
salt and freshly
ground black pepper

I always cook this traditional Provençal dish in large quantities so that I can freeze and reheat it as needed for a healthy meal (if you want to do the same, double the quantities given here). It is packed with phytochemicals like lycopene (from the tomatoes), vitamins A and C, potassium, fibres – and has virtually no cholesterol or saturated fat. A good example of a Mediterranean-diet recipe! You will need a heavy-based casserole for this dish.

1   Wash all the vegetables and herbs. Do not peel the vegetables.

2   Chop the tomatoes, courgettes and aubergines into 2cm-pieces.

3   Finely slice the peppers (remove all seeds as they have a bitter taste).

4   Slice the onions and finely chop the garlic and herbs. In a small saucepan, gently cook the onion in 1 tbsp olive oil over a low heat, until brown (about 15 minutes).

5   In a large casserole, heat ½ tbsp olive oil and sauté the tomatoes over medium heat for about 10 minutes. Set aside and keep them warm. Sauté the courgettes in a little more olive oil until browned and tender. Set aside with the tomatoes.

6   Repeat the process with the peppers, the aubergines and garlic.

7   Mix all the cooked ingredients, add the chopped herbs and cook on low for at least 30 minutes. If you can cook longer at very low temperature, the taste will be more intense.

8   Season to taste before serving. Can be served hot or cold.

YOGURT SAUCE

Serves 4
Preparation 5 min

Ingredients
225g plain, lactose-
free yogurt
dash of mustard or
horseradish sauce
salt and freshly
ground black pepper
oregano (fresh or
dried; optional)
2 tsp balsamic
vinegar

This sauce is a delicious dip for serving with steamed artichoke without the fat of a regular oil-and-vinegar dressing. It is a healthy source of protein, too.

1   Whip the yogurt with a balloon whisk.

2   Add mustard or horseradish.

3   Add salt and pepper, to taste (and oregano, if you wish). Mix.

4   Add the vinegar, mix again, and voilà!

Variation: add bits of goat's or sheep's blue cheese for a sauce with a salty, robust flavour.

RAITA

Serves 2
Preparation 10 min

Ingredients
3 plain, vegan
yogurts (soy, almond
or lactose-free)
salt, to taste
bunch of fresh
coriander, leaves
finely chopped
(or 1 tsp dried)
4 tsp finely
chopped mint
1 cucumber,
peeled and diced

The cool cucumber in this lovely yogurt sauce makes a great contrast to spicy Indian dishes, such as Chicken Tandoori (p. 86). It's also yummy as a low-fat dip for carrot and celery sticks.

1   In a bowl, whisk the yogurt until smooth.

2   Add the salt and coriander.

3   Add the mint and diced cucumber and mix together gently with a spoon. Serve.

SOYANNAISE

Serves 5
Preparation 10 min

Ingredients
250g tofu (soft
or silken)
1½ tbsp lemon juice
1 tsp Dijon mustard
1 tsp cider vinegar
1 tsp sugar
salt and freshly
ground black pepper
7 tbsp sunflower oil

Here is a lighter mayonnaise, which works as a perfect substitute for regular mayonnaise. Eat light, eat wisely, eat healthy! You'll find soyannaise in the organic food aisle of most supermarkets. You can also make other dressings using this 'tofu mayonnaise' as your base. This will keep for one week in the fridge.

1   Blend the tofu, lemon juice, mustard, vinegar, sugar, salt and pepper in a mixer on high speed.

2   Add the sunflower oil gradually, until you have a smooth, homogeneous cream.

3   Store in the refrigerator in a jar.

Variation: make a curry Soyannaise dressing by combining 3 tbsp Soyannaise with 1 tbsp canola oil, plus a pinch of sea salt and 1 tsp curry powder, or according to taste. Delicious with leftover roast chicken and salad leaves.

SIX VINAIGRETTES

All serve 2-4

BALSAMIC VINAIGRETTE

Ingredients

1 tbsp Dijon mustard

1 tbsp balsamic vinegar

1 shallot, finely chopped

salt and freshly ground black pepper

2 tbsp canola oil

1   Whisk together the mustard, vinegar, shallot and salt. Leave to stand to allow the flavours to develop.

2   Add the oil and whisk again, then season to taste with pepper and a little more salt.

CHINESE VINAIGRETTE

Ingredients

4 tbsp rice vinegar

6 tbsp canola oil

1 tsp sesame oil (optional)

1 tbsp Soyannaise (p. 81)

salt and freshly ground black pepper

1   Whisk together the vinegar, oils and Soyannaise, or blend them in a blender.

2   Season to taste with salt and pepper.

GARLIC VINAIGRETTE

Ingredients

1 tbsp Dijon mustard

1 garlic clove, crushed

1 tbsp sherry vinegar

salt and freshly ground black pepper

3 tbsp olive oil

1   Whisk together the mustard, garlic, vinegar and salt. Leave to stand to allow the flavours to develop.

2   Add the olive oil and whisk again, then season to taste with pepper and a little more salt.

LEMON VINAIGRETTE

Ingredients
1 tbsp Dijon mustard
2 tbsp onion, finely chopped
1 tbsp white wine vinegar
1 tbsp lemon juice
salt and freshly ground black pepper
3 tbsp olive oil
small piece lemongrass, finely chopped (optional)

1   Whisk together the mustard, onion, vinegar, lemon juice and salt. I don't use a blender here, as I prefer to keep the chopped onion whole. Leave to stand to allow the flavours to develop.

2   Whisk in the olive oil and a few pieces of lemongrass, if liked, and mix well. Season to taste with pepper and a little more salt.

MIMOSA CHAMPAGNE VINAIGRETTE

Ingredients
1 tbsp Dijon mustard
2 tbsp onion, finely chopped
2 tbsp orange juice
2 tbsp champagne (or sparkling wine)
salt and white pepper
2 tbsp canola oil

1   Whisk together the mustard, onion, orange juice, champagne or sparkling wine and salt. Leave to stand to allow the flavours to develop.

2   Whisk in the canola oil, and season to taste with salt and white pepper. If you want a smooth texture, whizz in a blender.

SWEET SHALLOT VINAIGRETTE

Ingredients
1 tbsp coarse-grain mustard
1 shallot, finely chopped
1 tbsp aged balsamic vinegar
salt and freshly ground black pepper
3 tbsp canola oil

1   Whisk together the mustard, shallot, vinegar and salt. Leave to stand to allow the flavours to develop.

2   Add the canola oil and whisk again, then season to taste with pepper and a little more salt.

AVOCADO AND SALMON TORTILLA

Serves 1
Preparation 5 min

Ingredients
1 sprouted-grain or
wholewheat tortilla
1 tsp Soyannaise
(page 81; to help
keep the saturated
fat at zero)
½ ripe avocado,
peeled and sliced
lemon juice
100g wild smoked
salmon

Avocado is proven to lower cholesterol
and salmon, like avocado, provides healthy
fats (omega-6), which also contribute to
the lowering of cholesterol. You can find
sprouted-grain tortillas at good healthfood
shops and online, or substitute with
wholewheat if you're not in the DETOX phase.

1   Warm the tortilla in a hot, dry frying pan
for 1 minute on each side.

2   Place the tortilla on a plate.

3   Spread the Soyannaise over and scatter
with the slices of avocado. Drizzle over a
few drops of lemon juice.

4   Top with the salmon slices, adding a tiny
bit more lemon juice, if liked.

5   Fold in the ends and wrap up your filling.

SMOKED SALMON ROLLS WITH CREAM CHEESE

Serves 2
Preparation 10 min

Ingredients
75g fat-free, vegan
cream cheese
½ tsp chives,
finely chopped
salt, freshly ground
black pepper and
garlic powder, to
taste
4 slices smoked
salmon

This recipe is perfect as an appetiser or a
first course, and can be made in advance,
as it freezes very well. The salmon is rich in
protein and good fats. I like to serve these
rolls with berries, which are a good source
of antioxidants.

1   In a small bowl, use a fork to mix the
cream cheese, chives, salt, pepper and
garlic powder, to taste.

2   On a plate, lay one slice of smoked
salmon. Carefully spoon the cream-cheese
mixture evenly across the whole slice. Roll
up the slice as you would for a spring roll.
Repeat for the remaining slices.

3   Refrigerate until ready to eat. You can
slice the rolls to make smaller portions,
if you're serving them as an appetiser or
a first course.

TROUT FILLET IN HAZELNUT CRUST

Serves 1
Preparation 15 min

Ingredients
1 handful hazelnuts
(or almonds, if you
prefer)
1 trout fillet
(preferably wild, or
organically farmed)
1 tsp canola oil
lemon wedges,
to serve

This is delicious served simply with lemon wedges and a green salad for a light lunch. Add some brown basmati rice for a more substantial meal.

1   Wrap the hazelnuts or almonds in a clean tea towel and run a rolling pin over them to reduce to a coarse rubble. Transfer to a large plate.

2   Lay the trout fillet on the nuts and press to coat evenly. Turn over and repeat.

3   In a nonstick pan, heat the canola oil over a medium heat. Cook the trout fillet for about 3 minutes, then turn it over very carefully, keeping the nut crust in place as well as you can. Cook for another 3 minutes, or until done to your liking.

4   Serve with lemon wedges.

CHICKEN WITH LEMON AND CUMIN

Serves 2
Preparation 30 min

Ingredients
2 chicken breasts,
skin on
olive oil
sea salt, freshly
ground pepper
and cumin
½ lemon, thinly
sliced
8 pitted olives
(green or black)
2 garlic cloves

This mouth-watering chicken dish has beautiful, golden skin and a great flavour, thanks to the cumin. It's a good source of animal protein and is low in saturated fat. This recipe is easy to adapt for more people.

1   Brush the chicken breasts with olive oil. Sprinkle over salt, pepper and cumin. Transfer to an oiled oven dish, skin side uppermost.

2   Add the lemon, olives and garlic cloves. Bake for 30 minutes at 200°C/400°F/gas mark 6.

3   After 10 minutes, add 5 tbsp water, and do this twice more, every 5 minutes or so. If the chicken is looking dry, add a bit more water, but don't add too much or you'll end up with a watery sauce.

4   Serve with a green salad or steamed vegetables.

CHICKEN TANDOORI

Serves 2
Preparation 20 min,
plus marinading
time

This popular Indian dish is easy to make in your own home – you don't need to have a tandoori oven. You can remove the skin to cut back on calories and fat, if you prefer. I like to keep the skin on. This is delicious served with Raita yogurt sauce (p. 80).

Ingredients
2 chicken breasts
(on the bone or off),
or legs
pinch Kashmiri
red chilli powder,
or to taste
½ tsp lemon juice
salt, to taste

For the marinade
pinch red chilli
powder (my
preference is
Kashmiri red),
or to taste
salt, to taste
2 tsp grated ginger
2 large garlic cloves,
crushed
2 tsp lemon juice
½ tsp garam masala
powder
1 tsp mustard oil
60g plain soy yogurt
canola oil spray, if
using oven
2 tbsp melted butter
½ tsp chaat masala,
to serve
onion rings and
lemon wedges, to
garnish

1   Make incisions with a sharp knife all over the chicken.

2   Rub the chicken with a mixture of Kashmiri red chilli powder, lemon juice and salt. Cover and set aside in the fridge for half an hour.

3   To make the marinade, mix chilli powder, salt, ginger, garlic, lemon juice, garam masala powder and mustard oil with the yogurt.

4   Spread this marinade over the chicken pieces, cover and refrigerate for 3–4 hours (the longer, the better – so don't fret if you find you've left the chicken in the fridge for too long!).

5   If you're using a tandoor, prepare it to a moderate heat. Otherwise, preheat the oven to 200°C/400°F/gas mark 6. If using a tandoor, push the chicken onto the skewers and cook in the tandoor for 10-12 minutes, or until almost done. Chicken pieces with the bone in will take a little longer. If using an oven, simply spray or lightly grease a roasting dish with canola oil and bake for the same time, until golden. Turn the chicken pieces over halfway through so they are evenly roasted.

6   Baste with the melted butter and cook for another 4 minutes.

7   Sprinkle with chaat masala powder and serve with onion rings, lemon wedges and Raita, if liked.

FETA AND OLIVE PASTA SALAD

Serves 2
Preparation 10 min

Ingredients

120g cooked and refrigerated, or room-temperature gluten-free or wholewheat fusilli

8 pitted kalamata black olives, cut in half

5 (or to taste) basil leaves, rinsed, pat-dried and chopped

200g feta cheese, cubed

60ml olive oil, plus more, if needed

1 tbsp red wine vinegar

sea salt and freshly ground black pepper, to taste (keep in mind that feta cheese is salty, so make sure you taste before adding more salt!)

This is an interesting mix providing the vast majority of the nutrients we need for a meal: proteins, complex carbohydrates, dark leafy greens and so on. If you're making this recipe when you're not in the DETOX phase, replace the gluten-free pasta with wholewheat. This contains vitamin B6, which is critical for the absorption of magnesium. Feta cheese will provide you with indispensable protein and calcium. I use fusilli for this salad, as the feta cheese and other goodies get stuck in the twists!

1   Mix all the ingredients in a large salad bowl.

2   Serve immediately. (This is not a salad that can be kept for the following day as pasta will absorb the dressing and become mushy.)

Variations. I'm a blue-cheese lover, so I often add blue cheese to this salad. (Be aware that some blue cheeses are made with sheep's milk and others with cow's milk. Go for the sheep's milk version.)

SPINACH, STRAWBERRY AND APPLE SALAD

Serves 2
Preparation 10 min

Ingredients
Balsamic Vinaigrette (p. 82)
1 fresh bunch spinach, rinsed, drained, and pat-dried
40g dried strawberries, sliced
75g dried apple rings or half slices
salt and freshly ground black pepper

Spinach! This nutrient-rich, dark, leafy green provides calcium, magnesium, vitamin B6 and several other phytochemicals that seem to have excellent cancer-fighting properties, according to recent studies. Vitamin B6 is crucial for supporting your body's absorption of magnesium. A lack of magnesium can lead to a long list of health issues, including irritability, depression, insomnia, muscle weakness and cramps in the toes, feet, legs or fingers.

1   Prepare the vinaigrette.

2   Put the spinach in a large salad bowl. Add all but 1 tbsp of the vinaigrette.

3   Top with the dried strawberries and dried apples and drizzle the remaining dressing on top.

Variation: scatter over a tiny amount of sheep's blue cheese.

GRAPEFRUIT-STRAWBERRY MIX

Serves 2
Preparation 10 min

Ingredients
1 pink grapefruit, cut in half
140g strawberries, rinsed and cut in half
2 tsp orange-flower water
1 tsp granulated sugar or a little agave nectar

A colourful health boost and delicious palate-cleanser.

NOTE Pink grapefruit can interfere with some medications; check with your doctor first. Orange makes a good substitute.

1   Peel the grapefruit, keeping each half of the peel whole. Working over a bowl to collect the juices, use a paring knife to slice between each segment and its membrane. Remove the fruit and reserve the peel.

2   In a large bowl, toss the grapefruit sections with the reserved juice. Add the strawberries and orange-flower water. Mix.

3   Sprinkle over sugar or agave nectar, spoon into the grapefruit shells (or ramekins) and serve immediately.

TRI-COLOUR FRUIT SALAD

Serves 2
Preparation 15 min

Ingredients
250g strawberries
(fresh)
125g blueberries
(fresh or frozen)
250g raspberries
(fresh or frozen)
½ squeezed lemon
stevia
mint leaves, to
garnish

Enjoy the sweet freshness of berries, enhanced with the zing of lemon and the coolness of mint. Easy, delicious, healthy. In addition to folate, vitamin C, fibre and potassium, berries provide a high level of vitamin A, which helps maintain good vision, especially night vision. This salad is quick to prepare and provides powerful phytochemicals (such as flavonoids, with their anti-inflammatory properties), which will make your skin look great. In addition, berries are packed full of antioxidants, which provide protection by neutralising free radicals (harmful by-products of metabolism that can lead to cancer and other age-related diseases).

1   Rinse all the fresh berries. if using frozen, take them out of the freezer two hours before using them.

2   Cut the strawberries in half or in quarters, depending on size, and put them in a salad bowl.

3   Add the blueberries and mix.

4   Place half of the raspberries in a mixer and blend.

5   Add blended raspberries and whole raspberries to the fruit salad.

6   Add lemon juice and stir gently with a spoon.

7   Add stevia to taste. Decorate with mint leaves.

Variation: top with plain soy yogurt whipped with stevia.

ATTACK

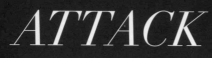

GOALS

Attack stubborn weight
and reduce cellulite

ATTACK

FACTS

- Glycaemic peaks make us fat.
- Yes, we can get rid of cellulite!

Rules of the ATTACK phase

- We do one TD Day per week.
- We drink Sobacha every morning, plus three cups throughout the day.
- We drink lemon juice with water every morning.
- We take one 30-minute walk on an empty stomach per day.
- We do one hour minimum of cardio per day, using this phase to try lots of different activities.
- We do two anti-cellulite exercises per day, plus as many '25th-hours' as we can fit in.
- We manage our stress with abdominal breathing exercises.

Congratulations! You have completed the first hurdle – the DETOX phase – and I am rooting for you! In the past 14 days you have cleansed your body and gently slimmed down all over. As you continue to get rid of toxins, your entire body is starting to look less bloated, you are experiencing a new level of vitality and, most importantly, you have lost your first pounds.

Your tummy is flatter; your clothes might even begin to feel a little bit looser all over. And, if you started out with a lot of weight to lose, you might even be considering buying jeans one-size down already!

Let's look at your success in numbers: check your weight first. Then, measure your waist, arms and thighs. Last, but not least, rate your energy levels. On a scale of one (no energy) to 10 (maximum energy), where would you say you are today?

The credit for these amazing results is ab-so-lute-ly all yours. So, obviously, you deserve a reward! (But not a biscuit or a big slice of cake!) How about some new exercise gear? A pair of super-cool walking shoes? Or you might prefer a spa treatment. Hey, your body has been put through its paces and deserves to be thanked, too.

Is the honeymoon nearing its end? We're often happy to push ourselves for two weeks, but then, our motivation tends to wane and we fall off the wagon. Not here! You are not alone and I'll be right with you every step of the way.

Instead of resting on our laurels, we're now going to step it up and put new techniques in place to tackle the stubborn weight that has become part of our life and has resisted even the most arduous of diets. We are going to, "Trash those pounds!" This extreme expression is actually the motto of an inspiring group of online BootCampers. I am honouring their community efforts here.

We're going to visualise those pounds removed, gone, expelled from our body; we are entering an **extreme-motivation** phase. Nobody, not even yourself, will get between you and your goal. And all your weight-loss saboteurs — co-workers who bring you a 4pm snack; friends who try to coax you into an extra glass of wine or the large pudding at a restaurant; the relative who gets upset if you don't have seconds – we're going to zone them all out. You're standing on solid ground and those stubborn pounds will melt thanks to the ATTACK phase.

Our goal is to consolidate your weight lost to date and continue on this path until you have lost 75 per cent of all the weight you want to drop.

Mind over matter
The mind is a powerful force when it comes to motivating yourself to lose weight. Visualisation techniques help you harness this power by focusing the mind on a memorable image. Here are three of my favourites:

1   **See yourself giving in**: a study from Carnegie Mellon University in Pennsylvania showed that visualising yourself eating a meal you crave can help you avoid binging. If you're contemplating eating a specific food you know isn't the best choice, try picturing yourself pigging out and enjoying the taste of the food, which could lessen your desire, or eliminate it completely.

2   **Know your 'enemy'**: when I am tired and lacking in motivation, I visualise an event in my life which is very stressful or a

person whom I wish to 'get rid of' (in figurative terms of course!), and it does wonders! I guarantee that such visualisations will give you enough motivation to go on that walk, do those exercises, lift that weight, say no to that cake!

3   Channel negative energy: for my Hollywood celebrities, I take another approach; I suggest that they think of the next casting call, of competing to get the part in their next movie. Or, if they've been left heartbroken from a relationship, I inspire them to channel their energy to get even more fit and beautiful than they were before; I call this the Vendetta Diet®. Again, it's all about harnessing energy and redirecting it towards something positive.

In short, each individual should tap into his/her specific source of motivation. There's no right or wrong, the choice is yours

LET'S ATTACK!

Now let's look at these key points of the ATTACK phase in more detail. Follow these rules carefully, referring back to my hints on 'extreme motivation', if you feel your spirit flagging.

1   One Turbo Detox Day (TD Day) per week

You have now become an expert at detoxifying your body, so let's use this knowledge in our ATTACK phase. Starting today, you will choose one day per week for your TD Day.

You might be wondering why you need to detox again so soon after the two-week, deep-cleansing DETOX phase. In the same way a house gets dirty with every day that passes, your body stacks toxins

– from stress, lack of sleep, some fast food that sneaks in here and there – with every passing hour. Remember: any change to our body WILL generate toxins. Even when we lose weight, our body produces toxins. So we are remaining vigilant and not letting any new toxic visitors put their feet under the table!

In a nutshell: we are constantly exposed to toxins so we need to have a cleansing schedule in place. That's where the TD Day comes in (see panel, opposite).

Make sure you stick to this weekly detox day. Don't skip it. But if you forget it, don't fret because you know that if you stress, you will only release more toxins and raise your level of cortisol. If you miss a TD Day, just do it the next day.

Invite your office colleagues to follow you in this challenge. Make it a game for your little ones who can pick and choose seven foods from the list, and motivate your other half to support you by doing the same and simultaneously doing good to his/her own body.

To maximise your chances of success, choose your TD Day now and write it down in your calendar, stick a note on the fridge and a Post-it in your bathroom. Put an alarm on your phone. This way, you simply cannot forget! And to ensure that you always have TD-Day foods available, keep a complete list of them in your handbag or up on your fridge, so that you are reminded to stay stocked.

After a few weeks you will be amazed at how natural and normal TD Days have become — so much so, that not only will you not forget about them, but on the rare occasions that you skip one, you will definitely feel like something is missing!

2   Sobacha every morning, plus three cups throughout the day

At your first taste of Sobacha (page 71), you might have been surprised by its unique flavour, but I am sure you've gradually become accustomed to it. Do you recognise all the benefits of this millennia-old drink? It's thanks to Sobacha that your appetite is under control and you are ingesting a high level of heart-and-blood-friendly antioxidants.

I have spent long hours corresponding with Chinese and Japanese internal medicine specialists about the benefits of infused, roasted buckwheat while sipping this wonder drink. I must admit that even I – your medical-study-obsessed coach – could not find any specific studies about the benefits of my beloved beverage. Why? Well, who would have any interest in funding studies on a readily available and affordable product that grows without pesticides? Not a pharmaceutical company, nor an industrial food manufacturer – both backers of many a study involving more valuable commodities or ingredients.

The best thing we can do is to look at how this plant has been consumed for over three thousand years – and at how you feel after having drunk it for the past two weeks or so. Even though I love proving everything I say with double blind studies conducted according to a strict protocol, in this particular case we have to base our decision to consume buokwheat on empirical studies (see also page 55).

Turbo Detox Day

1   In addition to abstaining from alcohol, gluten, yeast, eggs, rich sauces, sugar products and heavy foods (as for DETOX), stay away from all meat and all dairy.

2   On your designated TD Day you will consume **SEVEN** detox foods. Sounds too demanding? Not at all. Check out the list of 10 DETOX Foods (pp. 51–54).

Breakfast: freshly squeezed lemon juice in one cup room-temperature water, followed by Sobacha (p. 71) and Buckwheat Crêpes (p. 71).

Lunch: one steamed artichoke with Garlic Vinaigrette (p. 84), as part of a balanced meal of, say, grilled fish, then berries. That's five detox foods already!

Snacks: add an apple and a banana, and voilà!

For dinner, choose from the DETOX menu, or create your own healthy meal – but remember to stick to the rules in point 1. Of course, nothing prevents you from adding another TD Day when your body tells you, "I need it"!

Now that you know that lemon juice in room-temperature water does not give you heartburn – unless you suffer from specific medical conditions – I am sure you have become addicted! And that's great news. Your skin will glow more, your energy will hit high right from the start of the day and your liver functions stay strongly supported.

We are going to keep the morning-lemon-juice routine forever. Once again, you'll be surprised at how this has become a habit after just a few weeks. I am sure that if you miss a morning, you'll truly feel the need for it! So, make sure you always have some lemons handy (organic is great, but not mandatory) and stay away from pasteurised lemon juice because the heat from the pasteurisation process destroys vitamin C.

Do you feel ready? Are you mastering these three key components? I am sure that your answer is a resounding "YES!" So let's move on to another concept that is central to the ATTACK phase and to successful weight loss.

WEIGHT LOSS AND THE GLYCAEMIC INDEX

Studies on using the glycaemic index as a tool to lose weight were first published by the University of Toronto in 1981, based on the work of Dr Thomas Wolever and Dr David Jenkins, who were the first to study the impact of high-glycaemic-index foods on weight gain in great depth. Numerous independent studies have now confirmed those first reports and the concept is no longer contestable. It's crucial, then, that we absorb these findings and make them part of our weight-loss journey.

How can the glycaemic index help me lose weight?
If you have ever done a glycaemic test on an empty stomach you have witnessed first-hand what pure sugar does to your body. Remember that awful, very sugary drink the nurse gave you before taking blood? Remember how this made you feel nauseous? You are about to understand why!

Nutrition specialists have long recommended that we avoid sugars because of their molecular structure: simple carbohydrates (with a small, simple molecular structure) were labelled 'quick sugars' and accused of provoking a blood-sugar spike; complex carbs (with a complex structure) were defined as 'slow sugars' and prized for their capacity to satisfy our hunger in a sustained manner. Since the early 2000s, however, we've discovered that this classification is too simple and that simple carbs (carbs with small molecules) are not necessarily the only ones to be metabolised too fast. It seems some refined carbs with complex molecules (white rice and potato) also lead to a glycaemic spike, just like pure sugar.

This discovery is what led to a new kind of classification – 'the Glycaemic Index' – which takes into account the impact on blood sugar, regardless of the molecular structure of a food.

High-GI foods (with a GI close to 100) affect our blood sugar levels very rapidly. They are so quickly metabolised that they cause the body to store a lot of energy in the form of fat (glycogen). By provoking a glycaemic peak, or rise in blood sugar, followed by a brutal drop, they lead to cravings and fatigue. High-GI foods include: white sugar; white bread; steamed, boiled or baked potatoes, and sweets.

Low-GI foods (with a GI close to zero) affect our blood-sugar levels more slowly. They fill us up immediately and, by keeping our blood sugar low, keep us full for a long time, which means that less excess sugar is stored in the form of glycogen (fat). By preventing falls in blood sugar, low-GI foods help us fight cravings, stabilise our weight and protect against cardiovascular diseases and diabetes. Low-GI foods include: vegetables, pulses, meat and fish. Note that pure-fat foods like butter or oil contain no sugar at all and thus have no impact on our blood sugar.

You can see why it's so important to understand the glycaemic index of foods when trying to lose weight. Take my word for it – the proof will be on the scales!

Though the concept may be new to you, during the DETOX phase you've actually learned how to master your glycaemic levels without even knowing it. To help you get a better understanding of what low, medium, and high GI means, I've drawn up a simple table.

GLYCAEMIC INDEX	CATEGORY
<50	Low
Between 50 and 69	Medium
>70	High

What is the difference between the Glycaemic Index and the Glycaemic Load?

The Glycaemic Index (GI) is a measure of how quickly blood-glucose (i.e., blood sugar) levels rise after eating a particular type of food. Glucose has a glycaemic index of 100. The effects that different foods have on blood-sugar levels vary considerably. The Glycaemic Index estimates how much each gram of available carbohydrate (total carbohydrate minus fibre) in a food raises a person's blood-sugar level following consumption of the food, relative to consumption of pure glucose.

The Glycaemic Load (GL), invented by researchers at Harvard University, is more precise because the GI only takes into account the glucid (sugar, or carbohydrate) content of a food, while the GL takes into account the actual amount of *useable* carbohydrates, based on fibre and water content (fibre helps slow down the absorption of carbohydrates during digestion). This provides a more useful measure of the impact on our blood sugar, and hence on weight loss. That's why some foods can have a high GI but a low GL. For example, watermelon has a GI of 75 (high) but a GL of only five (low).

Here's a very simple guide to GL levels:

GLYCAEMIC LOAD	CATEGORY
<10	Low
Between 11 and 19	Medium
>20	High

Let's have a look at the formula which calculates GL.

FORMULA

Glycaemic Load = Glycaemic Index **x** (number of grams of glucids in one portion)/100

Now, let's see how we can apply this formula to calculate the GL of 100g each of watermelon and white rice.

Watermelon

The GI of watermelon is 75 (high) and one portion of 100g contains 6.5g glucids. So, to calculate the GL, we multiply 75 by 6.5 and divide by 100 (75 **x** 6.5/100 = 5). The answer is 5, which shows us that watermelon has a low GL.

Compare this with:

White rice
The GI of white rice is 80 (high) and one 100g portion contains 29g glucids. So, to calculate the GL, we multiply 80 by 29 and divide by 100 (80 x 29/100 = 23). The answer is 23, which shows us that white rice has a high GL.

Note that, although watermelon is known for having a high GI, it actually has a low GL (whereas white rice is high in both categories). This means that, thanks to the research on GL, diabetics can now enjoy watermelon – a fruit that was previously forbidden. The Glycaemic Load is thus a more complete indicator since it takes into account more elements than the Glycaemic Index.

Try it yourself!
1   What is the GL of a biscuit that has a GI of 75 and contains 75g of glucids for a 100g portion?

2   What is the GL of mashed potatoes that has a GI of 90 and contains 14g of glucids for a 100g portion? (Answers at the bottom of the page).

GL and cooking methods
Not only does the GL take into account the different components of a food but also the way it is cooked. Take a simple potato. When it is made into chips, its GI is 75 and its GL is 33 (both high), but when it is steamed, its GI is 65 and its GL only 14 (both medium). Why this difference? Because chips are more concentrated in glucids, due to water loss during the cooking process.

So, during the ATTACK phase, we are going to rely on GL to assess the foods we eat. This will help you lose weight quickly and efficiently because you'll understand better the impact food has on your weight. You'll be equipped with all the knowledge you need to create healthy, yummy meals which won't upset the equilibrium of your blood-sugar levels and will sustain durable, healthy weight loss.

Answers: Q1 = 56.25/high; Q2= 13/medium

ATTACK guide to GI/GL of common foods

	GI	GL
ANIMAL PROTEIN		
All meat, fish and seafood	0	0
Eggs	0	0
DAIRY		
Butter	0	0
Cheese (cow, sheep and goat)	0	0
Plain yogurts	36	2
Fruit yogurts	45	5
FRUITS		
Apples	29	5
Avocados	10	0.1
Bananas	60	12
Grapes	44	5
Kiwis	52	6
Mangoes	50	8
Melons	60	4
Oranges	42	4
Papaya	58	10
Pears	44	7
Raspberries	25	1
Strawberries	24	1
Tomatoes	15	1
Watermelons	72	4
Dried fruits: apricots/prunes	30	24
Dried fruits: dates	103	71
Dried fruits: grapes/figs	65	38
VEGETABLES AND PULSES		
Leafy greens (spinach, salad leaves)	15	1
Broccoli	13	1
Carrots (raw)	16	–
Carrots (cooked)	47	4.5
Green beans	30	1
Kale	10	1
Peas (fresh)	40	4
Steamed/boiled potato	65	14
Mashed potato	90	13
Baked potato	95	24

	GI	GL
VEGETABLES AND PULSES continued		
Sweet potato	50	10
Crisps	80	39
Chips	90	48
Pulses (chickpeas, lentils)	22	4
Hummus	54	7
GRAINS, CEREALS, NUTS AND SEEDS		
Buckwheat	50	15
Couscous	65	15
Quinoa	33	15
Wholewheat pasta (al dente)	49	9
Durum wheat pasta (al dente)	45	11
White rice	60	14
Basmati rice	50	12
Brown rice	50	12
Wholewheat bread	40	18
White bread	40	49
Dark rye bread	40	20
Pizza (margarita)	60	16
Porridge oats	58	13
Cornflakes	84	21
Muesli	56	10
DRINKS		
Apple juice	40	11
Orange juice	52	12
Fizzy drinks	63	17
Milk (low-fat and full-fat)	27	3
Vegan milk	36	6
PASTRIES AND SWEET STUFF		
Biscuits (such as shortbread)	52	16
Plain croissant	67	17
Dark chocolate bar	50	32
Milk chocolate bar	60	42
Jam	51	10
Rice pudding	56	23
STORECUPBOARD		
Spices (cumin, curry, paprika, etc)	0	0
Oil (olive, grapeseed, canola, etc)	0	0
Ketchup	55	0
SWEETENERS		
Agave nectar	25	18
Honey	90	72
White and brown sugar	70	70

BE STRONG!

I strongly suggest you do not move on to the last phase (MAINTENANCE) until you have shed 75 per cent of the weight you want to lose.

For instance, if you started with 5kg to lose, you can progress to the next phase once you have lost 3.75kg. And if you started with 20kg to lose, don't proceed to MAINTENANCE until you have lost 17kg.

I know how frustrating it can be not to shed more than 500g or 1kg per week when you have a lot to lose, especially if you are surrounded by friends who lose weight rapidly on dangerous and depriving diets. But remember that they have a problem – a big one! An unbalanced diet with lots of deprivation means a body that will avenge itself the very instant you take the slightest detour from the prescribed regimen.

So, BE STRONG. I am here all the way with you.

STAYING ON TRACK

The ATTACK phase has given you everything you need to lose that extra weight, slowly but surely. However, if you have more than 6kg to lose, you may need a little extra help. Follow my weekly challenges, below, and you'll stay motivated and on top of your game until you achieve your goal body. You can also set your own challenges or join our multiple groups on Facebook: www.facebook.com/groups/lebootcampdiet.

- One week without rice.
- One week with 15,000 steps per day, rain or shine.
- One week with a smoothie every day for breakfast.
- One week with 30 minutes extra cardio per day.
- One week trying new grains and seeds such as teff or fonio, instead of rice, pasta and so on.
- One week trying three new sports or exercises (such as bokwa or new zumba).
- One week with four cups of Sobacha per day (page 71).
- One week with three swimming sessions of at least one kilometre (at your own pace, even very slowly).
- One week with five 25th-hour exercises, done in the morning.
- One week with hot or cold soup for dinner every day.

TOP 10 WEIGHT-LOSS TIPS

1 I buy foods I don't 'like'

If you are, like me, a seriously insatiable gourmand; in other words, you cannot resist the temptations your house harbours, you need an infallible strategy so that you never fall prey to those traps that lurk in the cupboards.

My solution? When it comes to treats, I choose flavours I don't like when I shop (or bake) for my family. Ice-cream? Orange; the only ice-cream flavour I don't care for – but, luckily, my family loves! Cake? Coffee. I really don't like the taste of coffee.

You know by now that I am a true advocate of delicious food and would never miss an occasion to thrill my tastebuds. But, I want to do so on my terms, not by falling into hidden traps.

And you? Which tastes and flavours don't you like? From now on these will guide how you shop. Of course, this only works if your tastes are different from those of your family. If they aren't … don't buy treats in the first place!

2 I blog

To make sure I stay on the right path I keep a blog – a public one (myblog.lebootcamp.com) and a private, little one, where I jot down my weight, body fat, thigh circumference, waist, and so on. I encourage you to take your measurements regularly – you will be so pleased to see your results that this will make you happy!

I am frequently asked, "How often should I weigh myself?" There is no perfect rule but, apart from during DETOX where I suggest a daily weigh-in, I recommend you weigh yourself every week.

However, some people prefer to keep a tight rein on their weight. For them (and me) a daily morning weigh-in becomes part of our routine, just like brushing your teeth or taking a shower. As long as this does not become an obsession, you are fine.

3 I create a weight-loss photo album

Take pictures of yourself! This will do wonders if you have a lot of weight to lose. To make this experience as positive as possible, I suggest you take a picture each week, in the same place, in the same outfit.

At the end of your journey you will be able to create a surprising slideshow of your figure's evolution with time.

Make sure you take pictures of yourself from different angles (profile, face, back; zooming in on certain trouble zones) so as to fully appreciate your fantastic results down the line.

4 I exercise effortlessly thanks to my '25ᵗʰ-hour' exercises (see DETOX, pp. 46–49).

5 I use mint to suppress my appetite
This tip is totally empirical and stems from my personal experience, which I have shared with numerous BootCampers over the years. Chew mint-flavoured gum at the end of the meal, or brush your teeth with a mint toothpaste. You'll be amazed at how you are no longer attracted by this piece of cheesecake or that big brownie.

When you need to attend a party or function with a tempting buffet, arrive (discreetly) chewing mint gum so that you spend your first few minutes doing this instead of jumping on the rich foods. Empirical studies have shown that this tip can help you curb your appetite by 25 per cent. Don't forget to choose a chewing gum that does not contain toxic sweeteners (pp. 33–37).

6 I buy myself a nice piece of jewellery when I'm successful at losing weight
Do you love jewels? If the answer's, "Yes!" then give yourself a bracelet, a pendant, a necklace, a ring, or even a nice ribbon to tie around your wrist. It doesn't have to be expensive – it could come from the market, or be homemade. This will remind you of your weight-loss goals throughout the day.

If you need an extra prompt, choose a bracelet with charms that make a noise when you move. This noise will guarantee you keep your eyes on the prize: namely, your dream body!

7 I aim for one notch down on my belt
Write on the inside of your belt, "I want to get to this notch," with a little arrow. Of course, nobody will see this motivational statement but you. Make sure you do this for the next notch and the one after that … until you have reached your dream waist size.

8 Tea signals the end of the meal
If, like me, you like to end a meal on a sweet note, a square of chocolate, two spoonfuls of your companion's dessert (my favourite solution!) does the trick.

The problem is that we very rarely stop after those two spoonfuls because we are also tempted to finish the whole plate, to polish off our kids' desserts; and so on. Without realising it, we end up eating more than 200 calories. Remember that to produce one pound of fat you only need 3,500 excess calories; so at a rate of 200 calories per day, that would take only 17 days. Scary, isn't it?

A nice cup of tea is my absolute signal that the meal is over. And to help keep a flat tummy I usually go for an infusion of fresh mint (with no black or green tea added, and no milk), which reduces bloating

9 I leave my photo on the fridge

I often read in women's magazines that nothing beats the picture of a very overweight lady taped on the fridge door, to prevent you from opening it and gorging yourself. I have a radically opposite approach: if you constantly see an overweight person (you or somebody else) you'll soon begin thinking this is the new norm.

That's why I prefer to do the reverse: find a picture of yourself when you had your dream body, or choose a celeb or an unknown person whose body looks healthy and simply amazing. Then glue a cutout of your face on top of her body and place this picture on your fridge. Each time you lay eyes on this picture you will subconsciously think, "I want to look hot, too. I can do it!", or, "How about I go for a 30-minute walk?"

IMPORTANT NOTE: *please* don't go for an unhealthy, skinny girl, ok? Your goal should, first and foremost, to be the healthiest that *you* can be – I'm not suggesting you try and turn into someone else!

10 I never, ever, wait for the lift

The University of South Carolina Aiken has conducted an interesting study, which concludes that, since lifts always take some time to arrive, if you take the stairs instead you will gain an average of 20 seconds. (In this study, the stairs were within view of the lift).

This amusing finding points to one conclusion: save time, tone your thighs, mould your calves and slim your ankles by taking the stairs. Those 'gazelle legs' are within your reach!

CELLULITE AND WEIGHT LOSS

Now that we have put in place the nutrition part of this ATTACK phase, it is time to tackle one major project: cellulite eradication!

Getting rid of as much cellulite as possible is an important part of our weight-loss programme. What's the point in looking skinny in your bikini if your body is flabby? Together, we are going to take a three-pronged approach: tackle excess weight, tone muscles and improve the skin.

WHAT IS CELLULITE?

The official, medical definition of cellulite (also called superficial lipodystrophy, among other terms) is *'the herniation of subcutaneous fat within fibrous connective tissue that manifests topographically as skin dimpling and nodularity, often on the pelvic region (specifically the buttocks), lower limbs and abdomen'.*

In simple language, cellulite is a cluster of fat cells under the skin – which I like to call 'cottage-cheese skin', or 'orange-peel syndrome'.

WHERE CAN WE FIND CELLULITE?

You must have noticed that almost 100 per cent of the time, cellulite is a female problem. Indeed, 98 per cent of women suffer from cellulite compared with only 2 per cent of men! This is pretty normal, since its cause is linked to the female hormone, oestrogen. In women, cellulite is usually located in: the hips, thighs and abdomen.

HOW DOES CELLULITE FORM?

Cellulite can be caused by hormonal factors (water retention stemming from hyperoestrogenism that can come with menopause); genetics (blood flow, size of fat cells); and, very important, your lifestyle! Yo-yo dieting has been shown to aggravate cellulite, as does a high-stress lifestyle because it may lead to an increase in the level of catecholamines (neurotransmitters), which have been associated with the accumulation of cellulite.

But the good news is that certain dieting practices can diminish the level of these chemicals, and less body fat typically results in an improvement in the appearance of cellulite. A diet which steers clear of blood-sugar roller coasters – a low-GL diet – is ideal.

Why are we talking about the appearance of cellulite? Because a diet high in fat and sugar leads to the storage of lipids in fat cells called adipocytes. As time goes on the size of the adipocytes increases, which in turn leads to a thickening of the hypodermis (beneath the epidermis). The greater the lipid surplus (stored in the form of triglycerides), the more we notice a swelling of adipocytes as they fill up with fat – they can inflate up to 50 times their original size. Impressive isn't it?

In turn, this leads to a compression of the blood and lymph flow, and an inadequate drainage of water and toxins from the body. This accumulation of waste then causes a clustering of fat cells, making the skin look uneven and bumpy – that famous orange-peel syndrome. It's a vicious cycle that you alone can stop!

Furthermore, a lack of physical activity slows blood flow which means it can't drain toxins efficiently. Lack of exercise also affects muscle tone, making cellulite more visible. So, a larger woman who follows a balanced diet and regular, albeit gentle, physical activity will most likely have less cellulite than a thinner woman who is inactive and follows a poor diet.

Now you know that it is essential to move every day – without sweating it out for hours, true – but with consistency and regularity. At the end of this chapter we will review our fitness plan and look at some exercises that will help target our most problematic body zones and boost results (see pages 112–118).

HOW DO WE GET RID OF CELLULITE?

Diet: overhaul your diet by reducing your daily intake of calories, sugar and fat. Most importantly, put in place a low-glycaemic-load meal plan so that your body stores less fat. In short, follow LeBootCamp Diet!

Move!: ideally, by adopting endurance activities like walking, swimming or bike-riding. Even better, swimming in open waters will help massage your thighs and hips in ways that even a regular massage can't accomplish.

Massage: hand massages (with the focus on tissue stimulation, lymphatic drainage and motorised rolling techniques), or mechanical massages with contraptions like the Cellu M6® or VelaShape® (available in salons) are efficient, but of course, are no substitute for a healthy lifestyle. One of the more effective ways of improving the appearance of cellulite is dry-brushing: before showering, brush your skin with a loofah in long sweeping motions towards the heart. This will boost circulation and stimulate drainage of toxins.

Surgery and cosmetic procedures: mesotherapy and soy-protein injections are pretty popular in France and in the USA, for example, and have been tried by the vast majority of A-listers in Hollywood. However, some clinics carrying out these procedures use injections that have not been properly tested, and in some cases, terrible consequences, such as tissue necrosis (death of tissue), have been reported.

So, *do your homework first!* With regards to liposuction, note that while it will remove extra fat, it will not necessarily smooth out cellulite.

ATTACK PLAN against cellulite

Now that we know almost everything there is to know about cellulite, let's get going and attack these unsightly lumps on our tummy, bum, thighs and hips, in two key ways: a 30-minute walk on an empty stomach, and a targeted 'trouble-zone' exercise plan.

1   Thirty-minute walk on an empty stomach

Starting today, your primary goal is to walk a minimum of 30 minutes on an empty stomach, every morning. When I say 'empty stomach', I mean empty of solids – not liquids. Before you head out, drink your lemon juice in room-temperature water, followed by your Sobacha (page 71; as for DETOX). If you absolutely cannot walk 30 minutes on an empty stomach in the morning (it's too cold, too dark or an unsafe area; you've zero time; you're on a plane) then choose another time during the day, such as before lunch, snack or dinner – this should be four hours after a meal. I am sure you can find the time!

Ideally, we should add another 30 minutes to our walking time, to reach the sacrosanct standard of 10,000 steps per day (this is the amount agreed by medical professionals across the world. I prefer to push myself and aim for 11,000). There are lots of different, free mobile phone apps for measuring your steps. You build up the extra time in 15-minute chunks throughout the day, by walking to the station or the office, and so on.

Why on an empty stomach?
Several medical studies (Lariboisière Hospital, Paris in 2002; Kansas State University in 1995) have proven that you can lose weight effectively when you exercise on an empty stomach simply because you are using stored fat to expend the energy necessary to contract your muscles. These studies show that even if you burn the same calories for the same duration in both instances, when you exercise on an empty stomach you will burn 67 per cent of fat, as opposed to 50 per cent when you exercise on a non-empty stomach.

When exercising on an empty stomach, the body maintains stable blood-sugar levels by pumping out energy from fat stores throughout the body (from your 'saddlebags' for instance). This is because the primary fat store in our liver has been used up during the night to ensure our organs are nourished properly and to maintain a stable glycaemic level. This process is optimised when you perform moderate exercise on an empty stomach for a limited time.

WARNING The virtues of exercising on an empty stomach have been scientifically proven. However, practising any fitness routine on an empty stomach can have adverse effects if you go beyond 30 minutes, or if you push yourself too hard by going too fast. Since your own sugar reserves are limited, if you exercise with too much intensity you will make your body more toxic.

Indeed, if glucose is missing, our nerve cells will satisfy themselves with a replacement source of energy, called ketone bodies, produced by the degradation of fatty acids (lipids). When present in large quantities, ketone bodies become toxic waste for our body, potentially leading to kidney problems or poor recuperation. We will thus avoid all problems by settling for a leisurely morning walk.

Why walking is wonderful for weight loss

- Walking engages all muscle groups. While you walk, contract your abs to work your core, protect your back and tone your abdomen.
- A regular walk will greatly improve your cardiovascular health as well as your respiratory capacity.
- Walking does not strain your joints.
- The natural balancing of your arms allows your upper body to relax and your lungs to breathe better since there is no pressure on your chest.
- Walking helps increase bone density.
- Walking burns between 200 and 320 calories per hour.

- If you have a park nearby, a morning walk is an amazing opportunity to get some fresh air in your lungs, meditate in the great outdoors and super-charge your mind with positive thoughts.
- Walking is free and requires minimal equipment.

If the weather is not cooperating, if it is still dark, if your safety cannot be guaranteed or if you simply don't like to walk, you can also opt to ride a stationary bike for 30 minutes, go for a 30-minute swim, or any other sport that is not too intense. Choose what you like and what you will be most likely to stick to.

2   Targeted trouble-zone plan

It is proven that regular fitness activities like bike-riding or elliptical cross-training, combined with strength-training; or swimming and dancing, will help you tone up. However, it's only through targeted toning exercises that tackle flabbiness and cellulite, zone by zone (along with a balanced diet and a regular daily walk), that you'll achieve the body you dream of – and the one you deserve.

Together we are going to get rid of untoned abs, a saggy bum and thighs covered in cellulite. To see me perform the exercises that follow, go to www.lebootcamp/uk/exercises. Try and do at least two or three of these exercises a day, as a minimum.

LET'S TONE YOUR TUMMY!

For women, a tummy that's too toned is not necessarily attractive, but nor is a muffin top hanging over your jeans. We are going to find the right balance by practising easy but very efficient fitness routines *re-gu-lar-ly*. You WILL see results, but only if you lose weight at the same time: in order for your efforts to become truly visible your body fat must be below 25 per cent (you can use a bio-impedence scale or a body fat monitor for this. These are becoming more affordable and are available online and at some gyms). For your abdomen to be sexily toned, target the following zones:

1   TRANSVERSE

This muscle is invisible since it is under the rectus abdominis (the one that gives you the six-pack) and serves the purpose of supporting our internal organs. This is my favourite muscle to work on as it is the easiest!

- **Open the Door to a Flat Tummy:** we first covered this 25th-hour exercise in DETOX (page 48). Simply suck in your stomach every time you go through a door or hear the phone ring. No sweating necessary and results are guaranteed!

Cut the crunch!

Contrary to popular belief, abdominal muscles are amongst the easiest to tone and don't require a dedicated training session: 10 minutes per day is sufficient, even less if you are short on time. Above all, avoid hour-long abs or butt group classes which, too often, rely on the infamous 'crunch', where you push your reproductive organs down. Needless to say, this is not at all healthy for women. More and more gynaecologists are screaming, "Stop the massacre!", and with good reason, because they are noticing more and more prolapses in women who have practised too many ill-chosen ab moves. So we are getting toned – but slowly, in the right way.

2   RECTUS ABDOMINIS

• **The Plank**: this exercise is quick, strengthens your core (to help prevent back problems), tones your deep abs (for a flat belly), biceps and triceps and stabilises your entire body. Do this exercise on a gym mat or carpet, so as not to hurt your arms on a hard surface.

1 Lie on your front, resting on elbows, with hands locked together.
2 Straighten your legs and raise your body so that it is parallel to the ground. Support yourself with your elbows and the balls of your feet. Face the floor, keeping your neck and head in a straight line and contracting your abs to keep a straight back. Be mindful not to arch your back too much; this is the most common error that people make when they feel like giving up.
3 Hold for 15 seconds. Rest, and hold again for another 15 seconds.

Beginners: 2 series; 1-min, 30-sec rest between series.
Intermediate: 3 series; 1-min rest between series.
Advanced: 4 series; 45-sec rest between series.

3   OBLIQUES

These side muscles help define our waist. All side-ab exercises, or any which require a torsion of the torso, target the obliques.

• **The Boxer**: this is my all-time favourite exercise for obliques. It's very easy to do and does not require any specific equipment.

1 Stand straight, legs hip-width apart and slightly bent. Your back is straight and your abs are contracted.
2 Just like a boxer, you are going to cross punch: your right fist punches out towards the left, and your left fist punches towards the right of your body. Make rapid moves and keep your hips fixed and anchored. You should not be moving your hips or legs; the move comes from your core. You will very quickly feel how your obliques are engaged in this exercise!

Beginners: 2 series; 15 punches each side.
Intermediate: 3 series; 20 punches each side.
Advanced: 4 series; 30 punches each side.

> **TIP** Nothing prevents you (other than your neighbours!) from screaming with each punch to release excess negative energy.

LET'S SHAPE YOUR BUM!

It's very rare to hear women complain that their bum's too small! The problem is usually one of sagginess, which means our gluteal muscles need toning. Once again I have some easy exercises to give you a sexy, firm and peachy derrière in no time. You should already be doing 25th-hour exercises such as, 'Permanent Contraction' and 'Iron Butt' (DETOX, pages 48 and 47), whenever you can. To sculpt your bum even further I'll now introduce you to Lunges (page 116). This killer exercise targets all three gluteal muscles:

1   GLUTEUS MAXIMUS

If you are looking for the one muscle to blame for a saggy bum, this is it! Located behind the pelvis, it is the muscle that gives our derrière its round shape, so we will work it on a daily basis.

2   GLUTEUS MEDIUS

This is located on the side of our pelvis. It is a very important muscle as it defines the upper part of our buttocks. It is also known as the thigh abductor because it helps stabilise the pelvis when we stand on one leg.

How to lose 5kg in 30 seconds

I often practice what I call 'the Paris Hilton pose'. Look at her pictures: she always does the same sideways pose with her hands on her waist, tummy tucked in and chest out. We may not have the same figure as Paris, but there are ways to cheat the camera that we can all use. If you are conscious of your saddlebags, then put one hand on the side that is being photographed. This will 'erase' the excess fat on this trouble zone. Train in front of a mirror and you'll master this celeb pose in no time! Another great tip is to apply autobronzer on the skin that will be exposed for the photo – this really does make you look visibly thinner and more toned.

3   GLUTEUS MINIMUS

This is hidden beneath the Gluteus Medius, at hip level. It will get targeted every time you work on the other two gluteal muscles.

- **Lunges**
1 Stand straight, feet slightly apart, hands on hips. Engage your core abdominal muscles to stabilise your spine.
2 Step forward with your right foot, lifting only your left heel to allow you to advance as much as possible.
3 As you move into the lunge position, create a 45-degree angle with your right knee. Focus on a downward movement of your hips, making sure you keep your knee right above your ankle, pointing in the same direction as your toes to avoid injury.
4 During the movement, bend slightly forward at your hips, but keep your back straight.
5 To return to your initial standing position, firmly push off with the front leg, activating both your thighs and glutes.

Beginners: 3 series of 10 reps each side.
Intermediate: 4 series of 20 reps each side.
Advanced: 5 series of 30 reps each side.

> **TIP** *you can make this exercise more difficult and get better results by holding a weighted bar or dumbbells in your hands.*

- **Chair Bum Lift:** this exercise tones all the glute muscles. I do this at home (with a sturdy chair), or in the park (with a bench) when I walk my dog. You could also use the side of your bed or the sofa.

1 Lying on your back on the floor, with your bum up against the chair's front legs, put your right leg up on the seat of the chair. Grab the front legs with your hands to maintain balance and alignment.
2 Keeping your back straight, raise your left leg up to the ceiling (with foot flexed) by lifting your pelvis. You should feel a contraction right under your glutes; this is what is will tone and define this area.
3 Bring your body back to the starting position and change sides.

Beginners: 3 series of 25 reps each side, 90-sec rest between series.
Intermediate: 4 series of 35 reps each side, 1-min rest between series.
Advanced: 5 series of 50 reps each side, 45-sec rest between series.

> **TIP** Beathe! Exhale to lift your leg up; inhale to lower it.

LET'S SCULPT YOUR LEGS!

By following my healthy weight-loss programme, you are already eating well and exercising for 30 minutes every day, so your thighs should be getting leaner as the days pass. Now we simply need to tone and define those muscles that were previously hidden under a layer of fat, into gazelle-like legs!

(We won't worry about your calves as, thanks to our daily activities, they are already pretty toned and, if anything, we dream of making them smaller rather than larger.)

To tone our thighs evenly, we need to target three areas: the adductors (the inside of the thighs), the abductors (the outside of the thighs), and the quadriceps (the group of four muscles on top of the thighs). All of these exercises can be done from the comfort of your own home.

1 ADDUCTORS

• **Nutcracker**: this is very effective for toned inner thighs.

1 Using a gym mat or towel (or on the carpet), get into a comfortable position on your right side.
2 Using your arms to support yourself, bend your left leg over your outstretched right leg.
3 Now raise the right leg as if you wanted to crush something between your legs. Raise the leg slowly, so that you can really feel the muscle contraction in your inner thigh.
4 Hold the contraction for a moment at the top, and then lower your leg back to the starting position.

Beginners: 3 series of 15 reps each side.
Intermediate: 5 series of 15 reps each side.
Advanced: 5 series of 15 reps each side. Add small weights to your ankles (start with 500g, then move up to 1kg, even 2kg) to make the movement a little more challenging and to work your muscles even harder.

• **Gazelle Legs:** this is great for getting rid of saddlebags.

1 Using a gym mat, towel (or the carpet), find a comfortable position on your right side. Keep your core strong and don't arch your back.

2 Using your arms to support yourself, keep your upper body upright and very gently raise your left leg in a controlled movement. Keep your foot pointed like a dancer, or flex it to work your muscles differently.

3 Lower your leg gently, always remaining in control of the movement.

> **TIP** close your eyes when you do this exercise so that you can focus on feeling the muscle work and establish the muscle-brain connection, to engage muscles more fully. You can also do this movement in front of a mirror to make sure your position is perfect.

Beginners: 3 series of 25 reps each side.
Intermediate: 4 series of 35 reps each side.
Advanced: 5 series of 50 reps each side with 500g ankle weights, then move up to 1kg, even 2kg.

3   QUADRICEPS

This group of four muscles, at the top of the thighs, is even easier to tone than the adductors and abductors. But you know this, as you should already be doing my 25th-hour exercise: 'Bathroom squats' (DETOX, page 46). Here's another 25th-hour exercise – it's my favourite for toning the thighs.

• **Invisible Chair**
Do this 25th-hour exercise while waiting for the kettle to boil, in the lift, or with a Swiss Ball against the wall. Lean your back flat against a wall with your feet shoulder-width apart – roughly 30–40cm. Your heels should be 30–40cm from the wall. Slide down the wall until you look as if you're sitting on a chair. Your legs should be at a 90-degree angle. Make sure your back is flat and your knees don't go over your toes; otherwise, you may create unnecessary pressure in your knee joints. Hold for as long as you can (from 30 seconds to two minutes, or until the kettle boils, or lift doors open), then rest and repeat.

PLATEAUS AND BENCHMARKING

As I told you in the introduction, I had weight issues of my own, in a far-away past (well, not that far away!). Diet after diet, there was always that one thing that drove me crazy: the dreaded 'plateau'. I'm sure you have found the same.

You have been at it for weeks, sweating at the gym, rationing yourself and depriving yourself of a social life but you've got to a point where the scales show no sign of tipping in the right direction. Argh! So, what the heck? You might as well have that giant, steaming pizza or the whole tub of ice-cream. You're massively frustrated, and you'll get your revenge. Won't you?

This all happens for a reason: you have been tricked into believing that your weight will drop steadily should you follow the programme to the letter. When you realised your hard work was not paying off, you might have gone online and consulted blogs and forums, only to be told that you're not following the diet properly. Infuriating! And likely to have you wracking your brains to work out where you went wrong.

So why all this confusion? Because on top of being taunted by images of successful dieters, the message distilled to you is: 'You *will* lose two pounds a week'. You have been led to believe that weight loss is a steady curve. You are under the false impression that you HAVE to lose some every week, or else you are plateauing – and this is not acceptable.

Well, let me tell you something, you have been deceived! My numerous years of coaching thousands of women of all ages and sizes have led me to embrace plateaus. In fact, I welcome them, I ask for them, even. I have discovered what they are really about and how they form new points of reference for us to use. This is what I call 'benchmarking'.

WHAT IS A PLATEAU?

A plateau defines the moment in a weight-loss journey where the dieter stops losing weight even though she or he is still following a healthy diet and fitness regimen.

WHY DOES A PLATEAU OCCUR?

- You reduce your caloric intake. Since your body needs energy to function, it releases its stores of glycogen (fat contained in the liver and in the muscles). Because glycogen binds to water, when it gets burned by the body for energy it releases a large amount of water.
  This leads to a rapid weight drop.
- You feel happy about this and you might not watch your diet as well as when you started out. You might even scale down a little on your physical activity.
- Because your overall muscle mass has dropped (remember, glycogen is stored in the muscles), your metabolism slows down.
- Because you eat less, your metabolism slows down even more to conserve more energy.

At that point you burn exactly what you eat and you have hit a plateau.

Some people, very few, never hit a plateau. For them weight loss is linear. They are an exception to the rule. The average dieter *will* experience plateaus.

My willingness to embrace plateaus led to my theory of 'benchmarking', which has since been proven to be effective by real BootCampers.

WHAT DOES BENCHMARKING MEAN?

The original meaning of benchmark is, 'A measure used to judge the level of something'. But now I'm going to take this definition and apply it to weight loss.

We're going to take your plateau weight and use it as a benchmark, or reference point. Then, we're going to work on this plateau weight to trick your mind into thinking this is your new, heaviest weight ever.

To achieve this state of mind requires some work on your part. Decide consciously that, if it took you years to gain 10kg, or even 50kg, or more, it makes sense that your body needs time to re-adjust to a lighter self as you shed the pounds.

Embrace your plateau by thinking, "If my body resists now, it is because I have found what bothers it." In truth, your body and your mind will resist change. But we all know that change is welcome when it comes to our health, wellbeing and happiness. You need to congratulate yourself when you have reached this point since you have found your body's weak spot.

Remind yourself that your body is not a machine, but a gracious, elegant and very delicate organism, which might not respond to having its buttons pushed as if it were a robot. This is why your weight loss doesn't always follow a straight line.

HOW LONG SHOULD A PLATEAU LAST?

Based on my empirical experience, each plateau should last, in weeks, one quarter of what you have lost in weight:

- If you have lost 4kg before hitting a plateau then stabilise it during one week before moving to the BOOSTER phase (page 150).
- If you have lost 10kg before hitting a plateau then remain at this weight for two-and-a-half weeks before starting your BOOSTER.

I am not saying you should eat more to keep your weight at a plateau! If your weight loss is progressing, keep it that way, continue following the ATTACK programme and menus, and move on to MAINTENANCE (page 175) when you have lost 75 per cent of the weight you'd like to shed.

My benchmarking theory applies to those of us who, all things being equal, don't seem to be able to progress to the next level of weight loss and, of course, to those who need to lose more than a mere 2kg.

To stabilise your weight during the benchmarking process (or plateau), just keep on following my ATTACK menus and fitness routine (see 'Rules of the ATTACK phase', page 93), make sure you get adequate sleep and manage your stress as you have been doing so far.

While we are enjoying the plateau for what it does to our mind and body we also need to make sure it has not come about due to our lack of commitment to the programme. Take a moment to have a hard look at what you are doing and answer the following questions (to which the answers should be 'yes'):

Yummy nutrition

Am I sticking to my TDD every week?	yes	no
Am I following the ATTACK menus?	yes	no
Have I kept my portions the same size?	yes	no
Have I made sure not to put my body into 'resistance mode' by eating too little in the past (before starting LeBootCamp Diet)?	yes	no

Easy fitness

Am I doing my daily 30-minute walk on an empty stomach?	yes	no
Am I doing one hour of cardio per day?	yes	no
Am I doing five 25th-hour exercises every day?	yes	no
Am I doing two anti-cellulite exercises every day?	yes	no

Motivation

Am I still motivated to lose weight?	yes	no
Am I constantly identifying and eliminating weight-loss saboteurs?	yes	no
Am I writing in my blog every day?	yes	no
Am I sharing my success on social media?	yes	no

Stress and sleep

Am I sleeping enough?	yes	no
Am I practising abdominal breathing techniques?	yes	no
Am I getting enough daylight?	yes	no
Am I having enough fun in my life?	yes	no

Goodbye plateau, hello BOOSTER!

We love and welcome our plateaus because they guarantee a long-term result, but we should learn when to extract ourselves from the embrace! So that you avoid the trap of staying at your plateau weight forever, calculate the date that will signal the end of the flat part of your weight-loss curve, and the start of the BOOSTER phase, following my formula on page 121. This date can be written on your fridge, or on a Post-it note on your computer.

Write your BOOSTER starting date here: _____

TOP 10 THINGS NOT TO DO DURING A PLATEAU

1   Starve yourself

Yes, if you stop eating you will lose weight. But, you will also send your body into starvation mode in the process. This means that it will learn better how to store the few calories you ingest, slow down your metabolism and make it increasingly harder to lose weight.

2   Skip meals

Skipping meals because you are not hungry is one thing, skipping meals to reduce your daily calorie intake is a big no-no. By introducing frequent famine scares you send your body the message that this might become a permanent state, hence that the rate of your metabolism should be slowed down for your survival. As we've seen in point 1, this is not a healthy, sustainable weight-loss strategy.

3   Reduce portions to a bare minimum

Controlling your portions is one thing (and a healthy one at that), making them too small will, yet again, send your body in starvation mode.

4   Try another diet

Stay focused on our programme. I never said it was going to be miraculous. I did say, however, that you will learn to establish a healthy lifestyle and reclaim your body. Trust me. I have helped thousands of women. I know it is not always a walk in the park but stay committed. Stay focused. Eyes on the prize!

5   Binge eat

Feeling depressed when the scales are not your friend might send you diving right into a tub of ice-cream. This self-punishment is simply a way to attempt to justify your apparent lack of results.

Also keep in mind that it is not because the scales are not showing a smaller number that your body is not working for you. Enjoy the other changes to your body: you might not be losing weight but you might be toning your muscles and losing inches all over ...

Give yourself a pat on the back for all those subtle, yet important, changes.

6 Stop exercising

You may well feel down when you hit a plateau, but this doesn't mean that you should give up your fitness routine. On the contrary, you should get more exercise to keep your endorphin levels high.

7 Stay indoors

When things don't go quite the way we want them to, we want to burrow under the duvet. It is a normal animal reaction but not a healthy one. You need sun. You need to meet people. You need to keep your serotonin levels high, so enjoy life and celebrate the new you!

8 Dress sad

Plateauing means celebrating your new body; not getting depressed because you stopped losing weight for a short period of time. Reward yourself for the progress you've made with a new, colourful top, scarf or dress Say no to dull, bland, shapeless, slouchy clothes as long as this plateau lasts!

9 Dwell on past diets

You might be tempted to think that you are failing at my programme. That when you hit a plateau on a previous diet, you just switched to another diet where you began starving yourself – so, you ended up with the (false) impression that you had broken through the plateau. You are NOT failing. Full stop. It's important to be patient: it takes time to imprint a new reference point on your brain.

10 Surround yourself with whiners

Easy to whine when surrounded by whiners, isn't it? Well, don't! You have nothing to complain about. Maybe a friend or two might ask you how well you are doing, and this might make you feel bad. Maybe. But you are stronger than any negative comments that might come your way. Who has lost the weight? YOU!

You are totally in charge and responsible for your success. Explain to your friend that you are benchmarking. You'll soon feel like the smart one, educating others against yo-yo dieting. Doesn't it feel good?

And no matter what happens, remember this:

- **You are rewiring your brain.**
- **You are succeeding.**

Because, to arrive at a plateau you had to lose weight in the first place!

ATTACK MENUS

Here are two weeks of menus for the ATTACK phase, to inspire you to make the right choices. There are a few recipes you'll recognise from DETOX on the menu and, of course, I have added a few low-GL recipes to tantalise your tastebuds!

I've made some suggestions for choices when eating out, but visit any restaurant you prefer. Check out the menu online and find out which dishes might fit the ATTACK criteria (for low-GL foods, see pages 102 and 103). That way, you can enjoy your meal out with the confidence that you are not breaking any rules.

Along with favouring low-GL foods (organic, where possible), you should start each meal with vegetable or animal protein, such as turkey or hummus; or with fibre (kale salad, soup); and keep sweet things for the end of the meal. This greatly reduces the impact of any sugar in the food, meaning the body stores less in the form of fat.

From this phase on, unless you are doing a BOOSTER or TD Day, you may enjoy one glass of red wine per day (two, for men). Remember to drink three cups of Sobacha per day, in addition to your morning cup. Finally, even though I'm not suggesting you follow a gluten-free diet here, feel free to replace bread with its gluten-free version.

DAY 1

BREAKFAST	Juice of ½ lemon in 125ml room-temperature water
	1 cup Sobacha (p. 71)
	1 Buckwheat Crêpe (p. 71)
	1 plain, regular yogurt
	Feast: pink grapefruit (see p. 88) or orange
LUNCH	**Feast:** salad of grated carrots with a drizzle of lemon juice
	Roasted Quails with Cumin (p. 142)
	Mock Mash (p. 238), steamed baby carrots and shallots
	1 slice wholegrain rye bread
	Feast: watermelon
SNACK	**Feast:** apple
	Handful walnuts
DINNER	½ melon with parma ham
	Celeriac Root with Pears (p.145)
	1 slice toasted wholegrain bread
	Chocolate-cherry Fondue (p. 149)

DAY 2

BREAKFAST	Juice of ½ lemon in 125ml room-temperature water
	1 cup Sobacha (p. 71)
	1 Buckwheat Crêpe (p. 71)
	Feast: red berries
	1 medium glass Almond Milk (p. 137)
LUNCH	Salad of chicory with 3 tbsp chopped walnuts and Garlic Vinaigrette (p. 82)
	Wholewheat pasta with basil and steamed seasonal vegetables
	Feast: seasonal fruit salad
SNACK	Celery with Roquefort Cheese (p. 140)
DINNER	Green salad (lettuce, baby leaf, or any green leaf) with your choice of vinaigrette (p. 82)
	Plain omelette
	Feast: Ratatouille Provençale (p. 79)
	1 pear

DAY 3

BREAKFAST

Juice of ½ lemon in 125ml
room-temperature water
1 cup Sobacha (p. 71)
1 Buckwheat Crêpe (p. 71)
3 tbsp fruit compote (seasonal fruits cooked
gently with splash of water)
2 kiwis and 3 prunes

LUNCH

Salad of baby-leaf spinach, with apple,
red cabbage, artichoke hearts and Lemon
Vinaigrette (p. 83)
1 slice wholegrain bread
1 grilled vegetarian steak
2 dried figs

SNACK

10 raw almonds
Kiwi and banana smoothie (made with
Almond Milk, p. 137)

DINNER

Watercress leaves with Garlic Vinaigrette
(p. 82)
Feast: Brussels Sprouts with Green Tea
(p. 77)
2 small, grilled sardines with grilled tomato
and seasonal herbs
Feast: blueberries or other seasonal berries

DAY 4

BREAKFAST

Juice of ½ lemon in 125ml room-temperature water

1 cup Sobacha (p. 71)

1 bowl muesli (no added sugar) plus almonds, hazelnuts and a little soy milk

LUNCH

Steamed globe artichoke with your choice of vinaigrette (p. 82)

1 veal escalope with soy cream, wholegrain rice and peas (pan-fry veal in 1 tbsp canola oil; swirl cream around pan after cooking veal to mix with juices)

1 plain yogurt

SNACK

1 Buckwheat Crêpe, plus 4 squares chocolate (your favourite)

DINNER

1 slice Cherry Tomato and Goat's Cheese Flan (p. 140)

Salad of lamb's lettuce with vinaigrette of your choice (p. 82)

1 soy yogurt

DAY 5

BREAKFAST

Juice of ½ lemon in 125ml room-temperature water

1 cup Sobacha (p. 71)

1 Buckwheat Crêpe (p. 71) with 1 tbsp strawberry jam

Freshly squeezed orange juice (use 2 oranges)

LUNCH

1 portion Stuffed Mushrooms with Walnut Pesto (p. 146)

Feast: Tomato salad with fresh basil

1 piece feta cheese

SNACK

2 prunes

10 raw almonds

DINNER

Grilled Mackerel with Melon (p. 141)

Feast: pumpkin gratin (pumpkin or squash baked with topping of wholegrain breadcrumbs)

4 squares chocolate (your favourite)

DAY 6

BREAKFAST	Juice of ½ lemon in 125ml room-temperature water 1 cup Sobacha (p. 71) 1 Buckwheat Crêpe (p. 71) 1 Green Morning Boost (p. 75)
LUNCH	**Feast:** Red Cabbage Stir-fry (p. 146) 1 salmon steak with 5 heaped tbsp steamed bulgur wheat 1 soy yogurt
SNACK	1 handful hazelnuts 2 dried apricots
DINNER	Salad of sliced, cooked beetroot with Garlic Vinaigrette (p. 82) Wholegrain pasta with parmesan 5 tbsp cottage cheese and sliced kiwi

DAY 7

BREAKFAST	Juice of ½ lemon in 125ml room-temperature water 1 cup Sobacha (p. 71) 1 Buckwheat Crêpe (p. 71) ½ mashed avocado with pinch sea salt 1 orange
LUNCH	Green salad with Balsamic Vinaigrette (p. 82) 1 grilled beef burger with steamed broccoli, 1 tbsp olive oil and pinch sea salt 1 slice wholegrain bread **Feast:** pear
SNACK	5 Brazil nuts 1 banana
DINNER	**Feast:** salad of crudités (raw veggies) with Yogurt Sauce (p. 80) 1 steamed or baked potato with 1 tbsp olive oil 1 slice roast ham Îles Flottantes (p. 243)

DAY 8

BREAKFAST

Juice of ½ lemon in 125ml
room-temperature water
1 cup Sobacha (p. 71)
Small bowl (50g) unsweetened muesli
with 250ml Almond Milk (p. 137)
1 cup seasonal berries (around 125g)

LUNCH

Eat out: Japanese restaurant
Feast: miso soup
1 small portion edamame
6 nigiri sushi (avoiding tuna and swordfish)
green tea

SNACK

1 small wholewheat pitta bread
2 tbsp Hummus (p. 76)
4 squares chocolate (your favourite)

DINNER

Feast: Carrot and Ginger Soup (p. 138)
2 slices wholewheat bread
2 slices sheep's cheese
3 clementines

DAY 9

BREAKFAST

Juice of ½ lemon in 125ml
room-temperature water
1 cup Sobacha (p. 71)
1 slice toasted, wholewheat bread drizzled
with 1 tbsp olive oil, topped with 1 mashed,
ripe tomato and pinch Maldon salt

LUNCH

Eat out: On the go
Wholewheat veggie sandwich (your choice)
Feast: apple
4 squares chocolate (your favourite)

SNACK

1 pink grapefruit
10 raw almonds

DINNER

Carrots with Ginger and Soy (p. 144)
Steamed cod with a drizzle of olive oil
Salad of rocket with vinaigrette of your
choice (p. 82)
3 clementines

DAY 10

BREAKFAST	Juice of ½ lemon in 125ml room-temperature water
	1 cup Sobacha (p. 71)
	1 Raw Chocolate and Maca Smoothie (p. 138)
LUNCH	Raw Pad Thai (p. 233)
	Grilled halibut with 1 tbsp olive oil, seasoning and lemon
	1 orange
SNACK	20 raw almonds plus 2 dried apricots
DINNER	Caramelised Jerusalem Artichokes (p. 143)
	Baked sweet potato
	Feast: seasonal berries

DAY 11

BREAKFAST	Juice of ½ lemon in 125ml room-temperature water
	1 cup Sobacha (p. 71)
	1 Buckwheat Crêpe (p. 71)
	1 Green Morning Boost (p. 75)
LUNCH	**Eat out:** Indian buffet
	Lentil soup
	Sautéed tofu
	Sautéed veggies
	Feast: fruit salad
SNACK	10 hazelnuts
	1 banana
DINNER	Sesame Chicken Pasta (p. 142)
	Salad of baby spinach with Chinese Vinaigrette (p. 82)
	4 squares chocolate (your favourite)

DAY 12

BREAKFAST	Juice of ½ lemon in 125ml room-temperature water 1 cup Sobacha (p. 71) 1 Buckwheat Crêpe (p. 71) 2 tbsp agave nectar (to drizzle on the crêpe) **Feast:** oranges
LUNCH	**Feast:** Fennel and Pink Grapefruit Salad (p. 147) Grilled turkey breast 1 slice wholewheat bread 1 homemade biscuit (flapjack or shortbread; or buy a good-quality oatmeal one)
SNACK	1 plain, vegan yogurt 1 tbsp strawberry jam
DINNER	**Eat out:** Spanish restaurant **Feast:** gazpacho, or any cold soup of your choice Vegetable tapas ½ portion of flan (a typical Spanish dessert)

DAY 13

BREAKFAST	Juice of ½ lemon in 125ml room-temperature water 1 cup Sobacha (p. 71) 1 Buckwheat Crêpe (p. 71) 2 tbsp Banana Coconut Compote (p. 148)
LUNCH	Garden salad with Balsamic Vinaigrette (p. 82) 10 wholewheat cheese crackers 2 tbsp goat's cheese **Feast:** seasonal berries 4 squares chocolate (your favourite)
SNACK	1 Date Smoothie (p. 72)
DINNER	Homemade risotto (your favourite recipe; I use chicken stock and white wine. At the end, I stir in 1 tbsp non-hydrogenated butter and 2 tbsp parmesan cheese for 4 servings) 1 slice ham 1 orange

DAY 14

BREAKFAST

Juice of ½ lemon in 125ml
room-temperature water
1 cup Sobacha (p. 71)
1 small bowl buckwheat porridge with
1 tbsp raw, organic honey and 1 tbsp raisins

LUNCH

Mushroom Cappuccino (p. 139)
Feast: 1 mesclun salad (baby spinach,
lamb's lettuce, rocket)
4 squares chocolate (your favourite)

SNACK

1 small bowl berries, plus 10 raw almonds

DINNER

Feast: Vegetable Skewers (p. 141)
Rabbit with Honey (p. 142)
1 vegan yogurt

ATTACK RECIPES

ALMOND MILK

Serves 1
Preparation 5 min,
plus overnight
soaking

Ingredients
1 handful fresh
almonds, soaked
in water overnight
1 tsp vanilla extract
(or less, if you
prefer a less distinct
vanilla taste)
2 tbsp agave
nectar or raw,
organic honey

Here is a way to enjoy 'milk', without any of the concerns that come with dairy products (such as lactose-intolerance). Almond milk is easy to make and is a fantastic source of enzymes beneficial for your health. My son, who is a good test, adores it! If you don't have time to make this, organic almond milk is widely available in supermarkets. This will keep in the fridge, covered, for three days.

1   The night before, soak the almonds in a bowl of water. Make sure they are completely covered in water as they will expand overnight.

2   In the morning, drain and rinse the almonds. Put in the blender with 2-3 times their volume of water (or according to your taste).

3   Blend for 1 minute until the liquid turns white and milky.

4   Filter the milk through very fine filter paper in order to eliminate pulp. Discard the pulp (I keep the pulp to make raw snack bars, but that's another story!).

5   Add the vanilla extract and agave nectar or honey. Drink immediately to benefit from all the vitamins!

Variation: you can also add some fruit – a banana or some strawberries – to make a tasty morning smoothie.

RAW CHOCOLATE AND MACA SMOOTHIE

Serves 1
Preparation 5 min

Ingredients
250ml Almond Milk
(p. 137)
1 banana
½ tsp vanilla extract
1 tsp agave nectar
1 tbsp maca powder
(preferably organic)
1 tsp camu camu
(available in organic
health food stores)
1 tbsp raw chocolate
powder, or 80 per
cent dark chocolate,
finely chopped

In this recipe you can replace the raw chocolate with dark chocolate (80 per cent cocoa solids), and you could easily just leave out the camu camu and maca powder. Camu camu is a shrub found in the Amazonian rainforest. Compared with oranges, this powder provides 30–50 times more vitamin C, ten times more iron, three times more niacin, twice as much riboflavin, and 50 per cent more phosphorus. Maca is a root belonging to the radish family. It is packed with antioxidants and contains seven essential amino acids. In short, it is really good for us!

1   Put all the ingredients in the blender and pulse.

2   Pour into a serving glass and enjoy right away.

CARROT AND GINGER SOUP

Serves 4
Preparation 40 min

Ingredients
750g carrots
1 onion
2 tbsp olive oil
salt and freshly
ground black pepper
1 tsp ground ginger

This soup freezes very well, so you could make a large batch to save time.

1   Peel the carrots and onion, then grate them separately in a food processor, or by hand.

2   In a saucepan, heat the olive oil and sauté the grated carrots and onion together for 10 minutes.

3   Season with salt and pepper and add the ginger. Add 750ml water.

4   Simmer for 10-15 minutes, then purée with a hand blender.

5   Ladle into soup bowls and serve.

MUSHROOM CAPPUCCINO

This elegant soup looks very chic served in tall, glass mugs.

Serves 2
Preparation 1 hour 15 min

Ingredients
1 onion
½ tsp non-hydrogenated margarine
250g button mushrooms, sliced
juice of ¼ lemon
120ml white wine
salt and freshly ground black pepper
120ml whipping cream
250g mixed mushrooms (such as shiitake, cremini, portobello)
1 tbsp olive oil
fresh parsley, finely chopped

1   Slice the onion. Heat the margarine in a saucepan. Sauté the sliced onion until translucent.

2   Add the button mushrooms and the lemon juice. Sear for a few minutes.

3   Cover with 500ml water and the white wine.

4   Season lightly with salt and simmer for 1 hour on low heat.

5   Remove from heat and cool.

6   Pour the mixture into a food processor and purée until smooth. Pour back in a saucepan and add the whipping cream. Simmer until thickened. Set aside.

7   In a frying pan, sauté the mixed mushrooms in some olive oil. Season with salt and pepper and add half the chopped parsley.

8   Ladle the mushroom 'cappuccino' into two bowls and garnish with the sautéed mushrooms.

9   Sprinkle over the remaining chopped parsley and serve hot.

CELERY WITH ROQUEFORT CHEESE

Serves 1
Preparation 15 min

Ingredients

4 medium to large celery stalks (200g)
240g plain, low-fat yogurt
30g blue cheese (Roquefort, ideally)
salt and white pepper, to taste

You can serve this dish with grilled chicken or baked ham (trimmed of fat).

1   Finely slice the celery stalks and remove any strings, if necessary.

2   Blanch the celery slices in 2cm salted water for about 2-3 minutes (no more, in order to keep them crunchy). Drain and rinse under cold running water.

3   In a small bowl, mix the yogurt, blue cheese, salt and pepper until well combined.

4   Add the celery and toss.

CHERRY TOMATO AND GOAT'S CHEESE FLAN

Serves 4
Preparation 35 min

Ingredients

500g cherry tomatoes
140g goat's cheese
2 eggs
20g cornflour (2 tbsp)
240ml fat-free soy milk
240ml fat-free vegan whipping cream
salt and freshly ground black pepper
8 chives, finely chopped

This is incredibly easy and quick to make, and quantities could be increased for a family meal.

1   Preheat the oven to 180°C/350°F/gas mark 4 for 10 minutes. Rinse and wipe the tomatoes. Dice the goat's cheese.

2   In a medium-size baking dish, make a layer of tomatoes and goat's cheese.

3   In a bowl, whisk the eggs and the cornflour. Add the milk and whipping cream while whisking.

4   Pour the mixture over the tomatoes and cheese.

5   Sprinkle over some salt and pepper and bake in the oven for about 20 minutes.

6   Remove from the oven and sprinkle with the chives. Enjoy hot or cold.

GRILLED MACKEREL WITH MELON

Serves 4
Preparation 15 min

Ingredients
8 small mackerel fillets
1 tsp grated, fresh ginger; or
2 tsp ground ginger
salt, to taste
¼ cantaloupe or charentais melon
1 tbsp olive oil, for greasing the oven dish

This recipe might sound like a strange combination but it is actually a classic Corsican dish – extremely tasty and very healthy!

1   Preheat the oven to 250°C/475°F/gas mark 9.

2   Season the mackerel fillets with ginger and salt, inside and out.

3   Peel and cut the melon lengthwise into small slices (the same length as the fillets). Place the melon inside the centre of the fillets (skin outside, flesh inside) and secure in place using kitchen string or raffia.

4   Place the fillets in a small, oiled oven dish, with the open side uppermost. Bake for 5 minutes, then check that the fish is cooked. If not, add 2 minutes at a time, but no more than 4 minutes in total.

SESAME CHICKEN PASTA

Serves 4
Preparation 35 min

Ingredients
salt and freshly ground black pepper
225g wholewheat spaghetti
100g fresh green beans
olive oil
225g chicken breast, cut into cubes
1 garlic clove, chopped
½ red pepper, diced
1 tbsp sesame seeds

1   Fill a large saucepan with water, add a pinch of salt and bring to the boil. Add the spaghetti and cook for 10 minutes or until al dente. Halfway through the cooking time, add the green beans.

2   While the pasta and beans are cooking, heat a little olive oil in a frying pan and add the chicken breast, chopped garlic and diced red pepper.

3   Season with salt and pepper and add 1-2 tbsp pasta water. Add another tbsp water if the pan becomes dry. Cook for 15 minutes.

4   Drain the spaghetti and beans and return to the saucepan. Add the chicken mixture and sesame seeds to the spaghetti.

5   Return to the stove and heat gently for 3-4 minutes so that the pasta takes on the flavour of the sesame chicken. Serve hot.

ROASTED QUAILS WITH CUMIN

Serves 2
Preparation 40 min

Ingredients
4 quails, cleaned
olive oil
salt and freshly
ground black pepper
1–2 tsp ground
cumin, or to taste
4 garlic cloves,
unpeeled
pitted black olives

These are delicious served with your favourite roasted vegetable or with mashed potatoes made with olive oil or non hydrogenated margarine. For a really healthy alternative, you could also serve them with Mock Mash (p. 238).

1   Preheat the oven to 180°C/350°F/gas mark 4.

2   Rub the quails with olive oil and season with salt, pepper and cumin.

3   Place the quails in a roasting pan. Add the garlic cloves and as many pitted olives as you like.

4   Cook the quails for 20 to 30 minutes. Check often and add water if necessary. Spoon some of the liquid over the quails to keep them moist.

RABBIT WITH HONEY

Serves 2
Preparation 30 min,
plus marinading
time

Ingredients
1 tbsp raw, organic
honey
3½ tbsp lemon juice
3½ tbsp soy sauce
2 rabbit thighs
2 tbsp olive oil
1 onion, thinly sliced
salt and freshly
ground black pepper

If you can't source rabbit, you could use chicken thighs for this recipe.

1   To make the marinade, warm the honey over a low heat. Add the lemon juice and soy sauce and mix. Remove from the heat.

2   Place the rabbit thighs or chicken thighs in a dish and pour the marinade over. Cover with cling film and leave to marinate for a few hours in the fridge.

3   Heat the olive oil in a casserole dish and add the sliced onion. Place the thighs and marinade in the dish and season with salt and pepper.

4   Cook for 15-20 minutes over a low heat, regularly turning the thighs. Add a little water if necessary.

5   Serve right away with Mock Mash (p. 238) or steamed quinoa.

VEGETABLE SKEWERS

Serves 2
Preparation 25 min

Ingredients
250g courgettes
250g aubergines
1 red pepper
1 green pepper
3 small shallots
salt, freshly ground
black pepper
ground cumin
juice of 1 lemon
80ml olive oil, plus
extra for drizzling

Fill your meals with colour! This can be used as an accompaniment to fish, meat or simply brown rice.

1   Rinse the courgettes, aubergines and peppers and pat dry. Slice courgettes about 1cm thick. Deseed the peppers, then cut into 1cm-wide strips. Peel the shallots and keep them whole.

2   Put all the vegetables into a large salad bowl. Sprinkle over salt, pepper and cumin. Drizzle with the lemon juice and olive oil. Mix carefully to coat all the vegetables. Preheat the grill to medium.

3   Skewer the vegetables, alternating the colours. Grill, turning the skewers about every 3 minutes. The vegetables should remain crisp.

4   To serve, drizzle with more olive oil.

CARAMELISED JERUSALEM ARTICHOKES

Serves 4
Preparation 30 min

Ingredients
700g Jerusalem
artichokes
100g non-
hydrogenated
margarine
2 garlic cloves,
chopped
salt and freshly
ground black pepper
small bunch chives,
finely chopped

Rich in potassium, calcium and phosphorus, the Jerusalem artichoke also contains very few calories.

1   Peel the Jerusalem artichokes and slice thinly.

2   Heat the margarine in a sauté pan. Add the artichoke slices and cook until fork-tender, stirring occasionally to stop them from catching. Add the garlic and stir again.

3   Cover and add some water, if necessary. Season with salt and pepper.

4   When there is no more liquid left in the pan, check that the artichokes are tender. If not, add a little more water and cook gently for another minute or so.

5   Sprinkle with chives and serve hot.

CARROTS WITH GINGER AND SOY

Serves 2
Preparation
20-30 min

Ingredients
20ml olive oil
1½ garlic cloves
1 tsp grated,
fresh ginger
110g regular carrots
(preferably organic),
julienned (cut into
matchsticks)
110g yellow carrots
(preferably organic),
julienned
salt and freshly
ground black pepper
½ tsp ground cumin
1 tsp soy sauce
small bunch
flat-leaf parsley,
finely chopped

Make sure you use organic carrots here.
If you can't find yellow carrots, then just
use 220g regular ones.

1   Heat the olive oil in a sauté pan. Add the
garlic, ginger and carrots.

2   Mix well and season with salt, pepper
and cumin. Add the soy sauce.

3   Simmer gently for 15-20 minutes, adding
a little water and stirring regularly.

4   Serve garnished with chopped parsley.

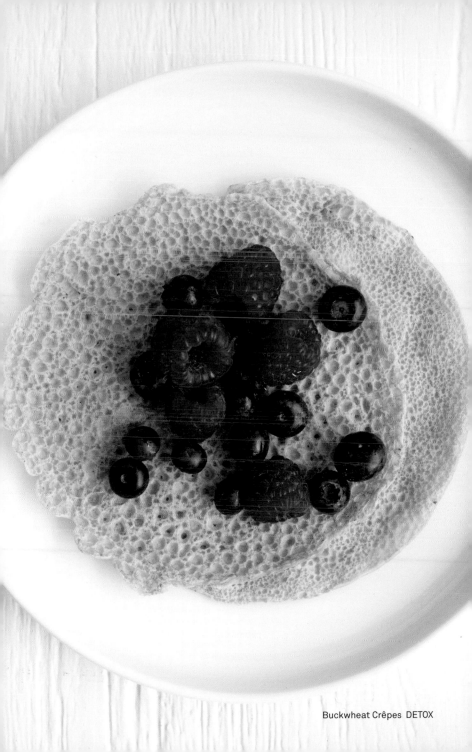

Buckwheat Crêpes DETOX

Provençale Ratatouille DETOX

Chicken Tandoori and Raita DETOX

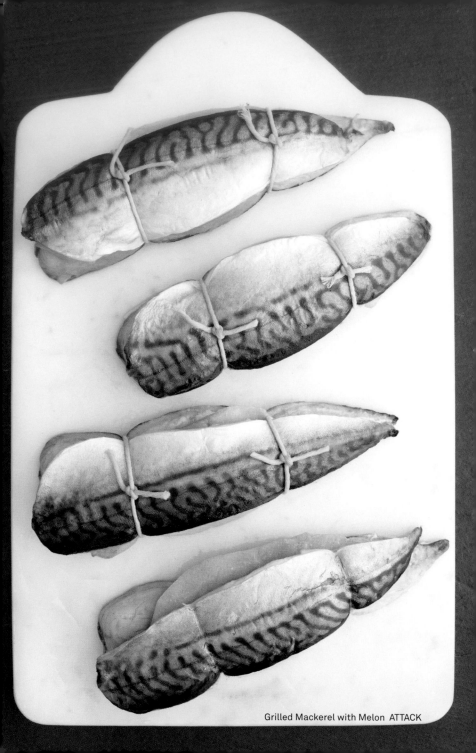

Grilled Mackerel with Melon ATTACK

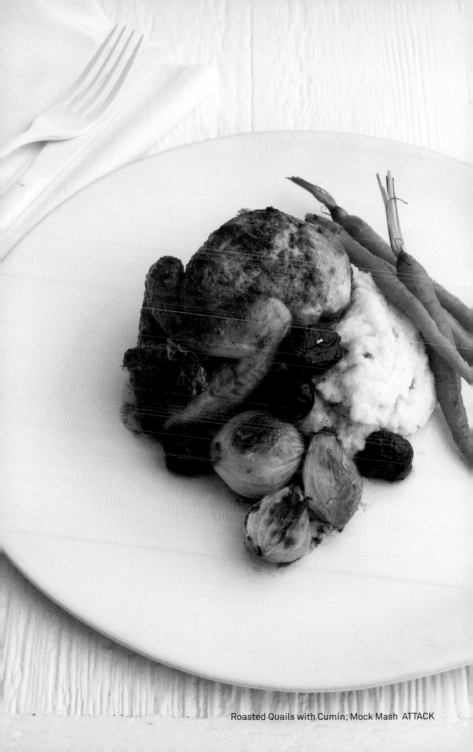

Roasted Quails with Cumin; Mock Mash ATTACK

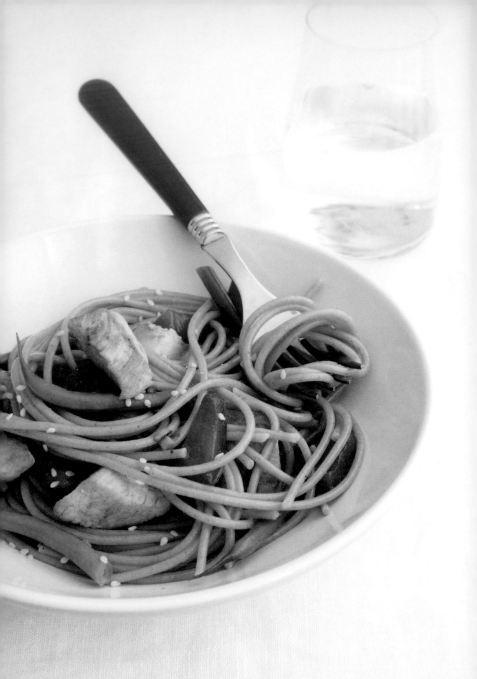

Sesame Chicken Pasta ATTACK

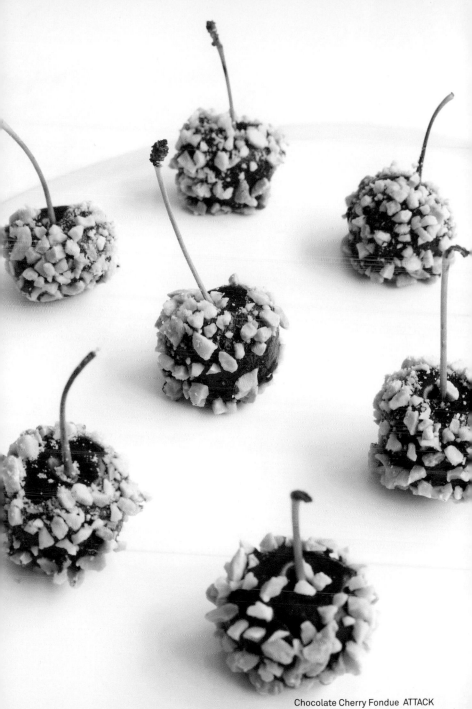

Chocolate Cherry Fondue ATTACK

Cherry Tomato and Goat's Cheese Flan ATTACK

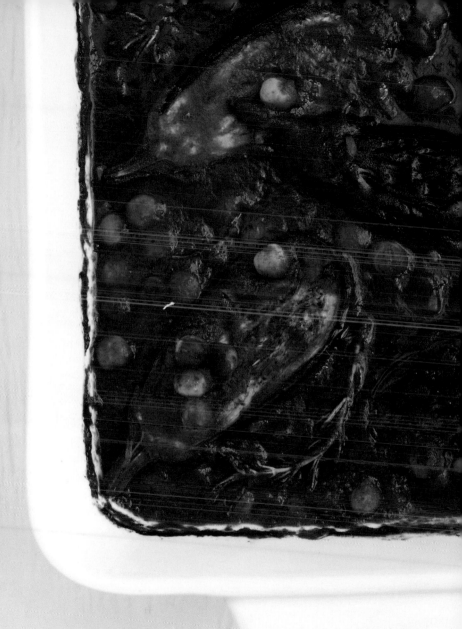

Italian Aubergines BOOSTER

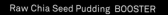
Raw Chia Seed Pudding BOOSTER

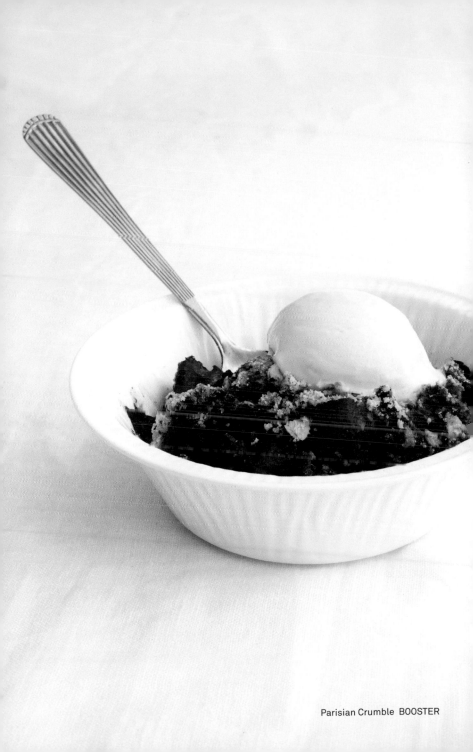

Parisian Crumble BOOSTER

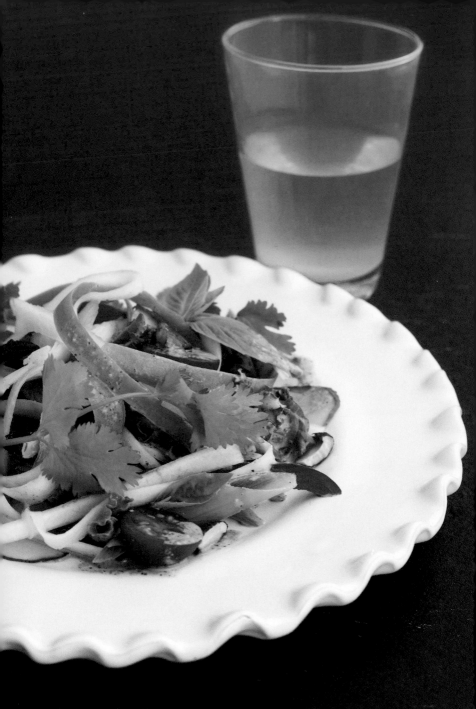

Raw Pad Thai MAINTENANCE

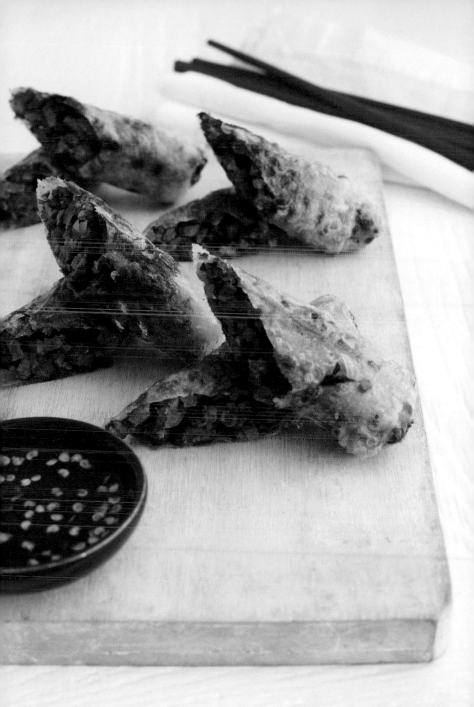

Beef Spring Rolls MAINTENANCE

Chilli con Carne MAINTENANCE

Chicory Boats with Smoked Salmon MAINTENANCE

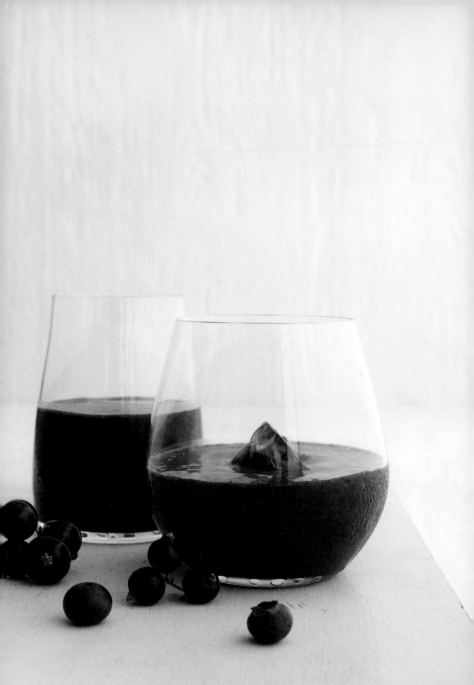

Purple Boost MAINTENANCE

CELERIAC WITH PEAR

Serves 2
Preparation 45 min

Ingredients
½ pear, unpeeled
½ large celeriac
(celery root)
juice of 1 lemon,
plus extra to
sprinkle over
celeriac
50g non-
hydrogenated
margarine
½ sprig fresh thyme
salt and freshly
ground black pepper

Celeriac is valuable in weight-loss diets, providing low-calorie fibre bulk, and is an excellent source of Vitamin C. For these reasons and more, it should be consumed regularly – not just once or twice a year.

As for pears, they are low in calories and contain a concentrated amount of essential nutrients: vitamins C, PP and B; potassium, calcium, magnesium, phosphorus, and zinc – an amazing contribution towards your daily recommended intake of vitamins and minerals!

1   Rinse and slice the pear. Brush the celeriac under running water, then peel it and cut into medium-sized slices. Drizzle the slices with lemon juice and toss to coat, to prevent any discolouration.

2   In a large frying pan, heat the margarine over low heat, then add the celeriac and pear slices. Add the thyme and half the lemon juice. Cover and cook gently for 30 minutes, carefully turning the celeriac and pears from time to time, and checking that the pan is not too dry. If it is, add 2 tbsp water.

3   After 30 minutes, transfer the mixture to a warmed serving dish.

4   In the same pan, over low heat, add the other half of the lemon juice and scrape the bits from the sides until the liquid is reduced. Drizzle over the celeriac and pear mixture, season to taste and serve.

RED CABBAGE STIR-FRY

Serves 2
Preparation 30 min

Ingredients
1 red cabbage
1 onion
6 button mushrooms
4 tbsp non-hydrogenated margarine
250g sweetcorn
1 pinch cinnamon
1 pinch ground cloves
1 pinch ground nutmeg
1 litre green tea
salt and freshly ground black pepper
3 spring onions

Enjoy cruciferous vegetables, like cabbage and Brussels sprouts as often as possible as they play a key role in detoxifying the body (remember that we still have one Turbo Detox Day per week in ATTACK).

1   Finely slice the red cabbage, onion and mushrooms.

2   In a large non-stick pan, sauté the onion and mushrooms in the margarine until golden brown. Add the cabbage. Cook for 10 minutes over medium heat, stirring every so often.

2   Add the sweetcorn (fresh or frozen), spices and 500ml green tea.

3   Stir and as the liquid evaporates, add the rest of the green tea to the pan.

4   When the cabbage is tender, season and transfer to a warmed serving dish. Finely chop the spring onions and sprinkle over.

STUFFED MUSHROOMS WITH WALNUT PESTO

Serves 2
Preparation 15 min, plus marinading

Ingredients
5 fresh mushrooms (crimini, or others)
5 tbsp olive oil
125ml soy sauce (reduced sodium)
125ml rice vinegar (or apple-cider vinegar)
salt and freshly ground black pepper
½ bunch basil leaves
5 walnuts
small handful pine nuts

A unique, raw-food dish, where all the nutrients of the ingredients are preserved. This is great as a starter, or a garnish to go with a main course (kids love it, too!).

1   Remove the caps from the mushrooms and brush to clean.

2   Place the caps in a large bowl. Drizzle with half the oil, the soy sauce, vinegar and seasoning. Leave to marinate for about 1 hour, stirring as often as you pass by the bowl.

3   Make the pesto. Put the basil, walnuts, pine nuts, the remaining oil and a pinch of salt and pepper in a food processor. Purée to achieve the consistency you prefer. I like my pesto thicker, while some like it thinner.

4   When the mushrooms have marinaded for at least 2 hours (or even overnight), drain them, place upside-down in a serving dish and stuff with the pesto.

FENNEL AND PINK GRAPEFRUIT SALAD

Serves 2
Preparation 15 min

Ingredients
1 large fennel bulb
1 firm pink
grapefruit
1 tsp lemon juice
salt and freshly
ground black pepper
3 tbsp fruity olive oil
fresh flat leaf
parsley, finely
chopped

Fennel is rich in fibre and supports good intestinal health and digestion. It is also an excellent stimulant and can soothe rheumatism. Grapefruit is now known for promoting low cholesterol; in fact, eating one every day for a month may reduce cholesterol in the body by 10 per cent. Remember that pink grapefruit can interfere with some medications. Consult your doctor if in doubt. Orange makes a good substitute.

1   Rinse the fennel and slice thinly.

2   Peel the grapefruit with a sharp knife. Remove the membrane, separate into sections and remove the skin over a bowl, reserving the juice as you go, then place the grapefruit sections in a colander to collect any remaining juice.

3   Combine the fennel and grapefruit in a salad bowl.

4   Make a vinaigrette with 2 tbsp of the grapefruit juice, the lemon juice, salt, pepper and olive oil.

5   Drizzle over the salad and toss carefully to coat. Garnish with chopped parsley. Serve right away.

BANANA-COCONUT COMPOTE

Serves 4
Preparation 30 min

Ingredients

10 small Golden
Delicious apples

2 small, very ripe
bananas

125ml water

juice of 1 lemon

1 vanilla pod

3 tbsp grated
coconut,
unsweetened if
possible

1 tbsp raw, organic
thyme honey (or any
other raw, organic
honey)

Remember to use organic apples and bananas. This keeps for five days in the fridge – cover with a tight lid – and also freezes very well.

1   Peel the apples and cut into pieces. Put them in a saucepan.

2   Peel the bananas and slice them into the pan.

3   Add the water and lemon juice, then split open the vanilla pod and scrape out the seeds and pulp into the pan.

4   Add the coconut and honey and cook over a low flame until the apples are quite tender.

5   Crush with a fork and serve warm.

CHOCOLATE-CHERRY FONDUE

Serves 2-4
Preparation 40 min

Ingredients
100g raw almonds
100g dark or milk chocolate (as you prefer)
80ml Almond Milk (p. 137)
500g cherries (I prefer the dark, sweet ones)

This is so easy, and so delicious! You can vary the recipe with all types of fruit. I love using strawberries (but NEVER use frozen fruits). If you prefer, you can make these ahead of time and leave them to dry on greaseproof paper to serve at a party or as a dessert.

1   Preheat the oven to 150°C/300°F/gas mark 2.

2   Roast the almonds for 20 minutes. Crush them using a rolling pin or in a standing mixer until you have a coarse texture.

3   Place the chocolate and almond milk in a double boiler, or a heatproof bowl over a pan of gently simmering water, making sure that the bowl is not touching the water. Leave the chocolate to melt, stirring occasionally. Keep warm.

4   Wash the cherries, keeping their stem on, as this will look nicer.

5   Dip the cherries in the chocolate, then roll them in the coarse almonds and enjoy immediately while the chocolate is still soft.

BOOSTER

GOALS

Speed up weight loss
and get a flat stomach

BOOSTER

FACTS

- Even though we are doing our best, toxins creep back into our body. To put this right, we periodically need a seven-day deep cleanse that will reset everything so we can continue losing weight efficiently and healthily.
- It is possible to get a really flat stomach!

Rules of the BOOSTER phase

- We drink Sobacha every morning.
- We drink lemon juice with water every morning.
- We eliminate all food containing yeast, and incorporate yeast-busting foods into our diet.
- We avoid all foods as for DETOX, plus a few more.
- We keep up our fitness routine, as for ATTACK.
- We manage our stress with abdominal breathing exercises.

You did it! You completed the first two weeks of my programme, the DETOX, with dedication and good spirit. You proceeded with the ATTACK phase and its weekly TD Day, and established your first benchmark. You have now stabilised your weight and need to get out of your benchmarking period; or, you are done with ATTACK but would like to reset your body before starting MAINTENANCE.

To speed up the process we are going to carry out a seven-day BOOSTER phase. You might find this week the hardest of my programme because of the limitations in foods you can eat. The beauty of this phase, however, is that you decide on the precise day that you start your BOOSTER. Wait until you have the time to take care of yourself, and more time for food shopping and cooking because, yes, this phase requires time-investment. But, I assure you, the results will be worth your efforts!

Once you are in the MAINTENANCE phase, do the BOOSTER whenever you feel you have overindulged and want to get back on track, or if you would like to flatten your tummy. In any event, never do it more than once a month.

This seven-day phase will serve three purposes:

1   **Speed up weight loss:** you might wonder why you need to do a BOOSTER. You have already made so many changes. You are eating better, you are doing your weekly TD Day, you are exercising regularly to tone your body as well as eliminate more toxins. The fact is that, even with the lifestyle you are developing, you are still exposed to stress, pollution and junk food. And, guess what? Losing weight also produces toxins, which are released when your body breaks down fat stores.

2   **Shrink your waist:** this is the number-one concern of all women (and men) I have ever coached. We all want a flat stomach but sometimes, no matter what we do, we still have a little round tummy. You might think that, because of your body shape, you are doomed. You are not! This should be your go-to phase whenever you find your abdomen not flat enough for your liking.

3   **Help you end a benchmarking period** in the ATTACK phase.

In order to achieve these goals, we will start a seven-day nutrition programme to cleanse your body and whittle your middle, boosting your energy into the bargain. During DETOX we began to clean toxins from our body. Here we are going deeper, from cleaning to 'cleansing'. The 's'; stands for SUPER, as in super clean and SUPER flat!

First, let's examine how yeast can make it harder to reach the goal of a flat tummy, and how eliminating it from our diet can lessen bloating.

A FLAT STOMACH AND THE YEAST CONNECTION

A long time ago, when I was carrying excess weight, I read studies on how an overgrowth of yeast in the gastrointestinal tract could have a negative impact on the figure. I dismissed these, thinking they were not based on scientific proof. But, as the years passed, I took the time to do more research. And upon the discovery that candida (*Candida Albicans*) was a major culprit, I found a way to gain a flat tummy.

We need candida to live. It is present everywhere in and on our body. But when it overgrows in our gut as a result of our lifestyle, it leads to inflammations, infections (the dreaded 'yeast infection'), athlete's foot, itchy skin, mental fogginess, irritability – and bloating.

Together, we will target your candida levels to make the dream of a flat abdomen a reality. (Your levels should already be lower, thanks to LeBootCamp Diet, but with these new steps you will be truly impressed by the results!).

> NOTE very few double-blind studies have actually proven that there is a link between candida and a flat stomach. Most traditional or conventional medicine practitioners tend to dismiss yeast cures, such as the ones that follow. I have drawn my conclusions from interviews I conducted with complementary and alternative medicine (CAM) practitioners, integrative medicine doctors and naturopaths.

Just for once in this book I will ask you to make your own mind up. Read around the subject (I recommend *The Yeast Connection Handbook* by WG Crook, Square One Publishing, 2008; see also References, page 248). Try it out. Following my guidelines won't hurt you and you might even witness a miracle!

What is yeast and where do we find it?
Yeast is a one-celled organism belonging to the fungi (mushroom) family. Yeast can be our best friend or our enemy, depending on the strain and quantity we harbour or use.

There are many kinds of yeast, from the one we use in our baking, to those we use to make wine, whiskey and beer, or the supplement we favour for its high level of B vitamins. In nature, we can find yeast practically everywhere: in the soil, on plants, in water, on the skin of animals and human beings.

Like salt and sugar, yeast is ubiquitous in our food. It can be found in the vast majority of biscuits, brioches, breads, pizza, food supplements, drinks and sauces. Along with mushrooms, foods like celery also contain high levels of moulds or fungi.

What feeds candida?
Candida thrives on sugar, starch, moulds and other yeast strains. To put it simply, too much yeast in your gut can make you feel bloated. In the BOOSTER menus at the end of this chapter, we will make sure we do not eat any foods that might support candida growth.

Eight foods to beat candida

1 **Garlic**: a recent study by the University of Maryland Medical Center reports that candida-prone people may help avoid infections by eating more garlic. So, over the seven days of the BOOSTER phase, add one clove of crushed, raw garlic per day to your meals, where possible.

2 **Probiotics** such as those contained in kefir (cultured milk), for example. The live bacteria in the kefir and probiotic yogurt will crowd out the candida yeast and restore balance to your gut system.

3 **Swede**: one of the most potent anti-fungal foods you can find. Try it in vegetable soup, as chips (with unscented coconut oil), or mashed.

4 **Coconut oil**: touted as a miracle weight-loss supplement, this might not, in fact, be such a marvel of nature (some studies have shown evidence to the contrary) but it offers potent anti-fungal properties. It contains high levels of lauric acid and caprylic acid, which help prevent candida overgrowth, while supporting your immune system.

5 **Onions**: these offer anti-fungal, anti-parasitic and anti-bacterial properties. Ideally, you should have onions every day. If you fear for your breath, add some parsley to your dish to counter the smell.

6 **Lemon juice**: lemon juice has so many positive benefits that it's on the menu in every single phase of LeBootCamp Diet. In terms of fighting candida, lemon juice stimulates the peristaltic action of your colon, increasing the efficiency of your digestive system.

7 **Cruciferae**: we've seen that cruciferae are fantastic for detoxing (Foods to Feast On, pp. 51–54). They are also very useful in the BOOSTER phase, as all cruciferous vegetables (broccoli, cabbage, rocket) contain isothiocyanates – compounds containing sulphur and nitrogen – which attack candida. However, see point 6, opposite.

8 **Cloves**: these contain eugenol, an anti-fungal essential oil which is extremely effective when ingested.

Eight ways to beat bloating

1 **Chew, chew, chew**: the digestive process starts in our mouth, so, the more time we take over chewing, the more time our saliva and its digestive enzymes have to get working. When food arrives in the stomach half-chewed, larger food particles pass into the gastrointestinal tract, leading to bloating.

2 **No fizzy drinks of any sort**: the air contained in carbonated drinks can get trapped in our digestive system, causing bloating.

3 **No gum**: chewing-gum can cause us to swallow air, which can then get trapped in our stomach. However, gum can be an ally when you're trying not to overeat (Top Ten Weight Loss Tips, p. 105).

4 **Pass on the salt**: too much sodium can cause bloating, too. Watch out for processed and frozen foods that can contain more than 200 per cent of your maximum daily allowance. At home, cook without salt and add it, in small quantities, just before serving.

5 **Control your portions**: when we eat more than the size of our stomach (remember, it's the size of your fist), digestion takes longer and food ferments. So, try eating four small meals a day – even five, if this works for you. See also page 60.

6 **Beware of gassy foods** like beans or cruciferous vegetables, which can lead to bloating with some not-so-nice social consequences. Cruciferae are excellent for attacking candida, but if you react to them in this way, stay away or take natural anti-gas supplements.

7 **Peppermint or fresh mint tea**: my all-time favourite. Enjoy it during your meals or any time you feel bloated for quick relief.

8 **Don't drink while you eat**: this dilutes digestive enzymes, causing food to take longer to digest, leading to fermentation and bloating. Ayurvedic medicine practitioners suggest that you avoid cold drinks while eating. Try warm drinks like green tea instead.

You now have all you need to start your seven-day BOOSTER, which will help you get back on the weight-loss bandwagon while working on getting a flatter tummy.

FITNESS ROUTINE

During this phase you will keep up with your fitness routine, i.e., at least 30 minutes of slow-paced activity (walking or swimming) on an empty stomach, plus one hour of cardio, two anti-cellulite exercises (pages 110–118) and five 25th-hour exercises per day (pages 46–49).

Of course, feel free to add more as you should have enough energy to be really active.

STRESS AND MOTIVATION

Since stress can cause bloating because of the reasons we have explored in DETOX, it is critical that you practice some of the breathing exercises I shared with you (page 42), on a daily basis. I practice mine first thing in the morning so that I can start my day with a renewed sense of purpose and a minimal level of stress.

And as for motivation, make sure you weigh yourself on the morning of the first day of the BOOSTER as well as measuring the circumference of your waist. And then DO NOT MEASURE anything until the end of the seven days. On the morning of day eight, when you get back to your ATTACK or MAINTENANCE phase, you will get a lovely surprise; trust me on this!

So, are you ready? Let's do it!

BOOSTER
FOOD GUIDE

Foods to avoid

- All dairy
- Eggs
- All meat
- Gluten
- Yeast
- Alcohol
- Carnivorous and
  predatory fish
- Non-organic fruits
  and vegetables
- High-sugar fruits
- Any drink containing caffeine
- Fizzy drinks (regular and diet)
- Rich sauces and heavy foods
- Sugar products
- All foods containing
  high-fructose corn syrup
- Aspartame and other
  potentially unsafe chemical
  sweeteners (pp. 33–37)
- Fizzy drinks (whether regular
  or diet)
- Processed food products
  containing additives that
  may be harmful
- Processed biscuits, sweets,
  cakes and ready meals

Foods to feast on

In addition to the anti-candida
foods mentioned earlier (garlic,
probiotics, swede, coconut oil,
onions, lemon juice, cruciferae,
cloves), you're free to indulge in
the following:

- Seafood
- Wild, small fish
- Non-starchy vegetables
- Fermented foods like
  sauerkraut or kimchi
- Low-sugar fruits
- Non-glutinous grains
  and seeds (quinoa,
  buckwheat, teff, fonio)
- Herbs and spices
- Sobacha and herbal teas
- Fresh green juices

BOOSTER MENUS

Our BOOSTER phase lasts seven days. During this time we will focus on cutting down on foods that encourage candida growth, and on increasing foods that reduce it. We also bring in as many metabolism-boosting ingredients as we can, such as spices and ginger.

If you wish to expand my menu suggestions feel free to tap into the DETOX menus and recipes as long as you stick to our rules for the BOOSTER phase, namely: no gluten, no yeast, no dairy, no meat and no alcohol. I do, however, allow kefir (cultured yogurt drink) on some occasions, as it is excellent for beating candida.

DAY 1

BREAKFAST	Juice of ½ lemon in 125ml room-temperature water
	1 cup peppermint tea (fresh mint infusion, or teabag)
	Cinnamon Buckwheat Cream (p. 167)
LUNCH	Grilled wild salmon steak with 1 pinch cayenne pepper
	Swede and onion gratin (sliced, layered and baked with 1 tbsp non-hydrogenated margarine and seasoning)
	Probiotic yogurt (vegan)
SNACK	10 raw, sprouted almonds (p. 65) with 1 glass kefir (cultured yogurt drink)
	Cinnamon tea (shop-bought bag is fine)
DINNER	Gazpacho (use your favourite recipe)
	4 tbsp steamed quinoa with lemon juice
	Chicken breast rubbed with grated ginger and grilled
	Ginger tea (infusion of grated ginger and hot water)

DAY 2

BREAKFAST	Juice of ½ lemon in 125ml room-temperature water
	1 cup peppermint tea
	2 Buckwheat Crêpes (p. 71)
LUNCH	**Eat out:** 'Mexican Buffet' (or make at home)
	Layer beans of your choice with lettuce, salsa, chopped tomato and avocado or Guacamole (p. 170)
SNACK	Buckwheat Crêpe (p. 71)
	1 tbsp homemade Almond Butter (p. 225)
	Flat Tummy Boost (p. 172)
DINNER	Steamed seasonal veggies with grilled chicken, kaiso or wakame (seaweed) salad and 4 tbsp steamed quinoa
	Parisian Crumble (p. 171)
	Ginger tea

DAY 3

BREAKFAST

Juice of ½ lemon in 125ml
room-temperature water
1 cup peppermint tea
Linseed porridge (p. 167)

LUNCH

Pissaladière with anchovies (bake Chickpea
Pie Crust, p. 173. Top with caramelised
onions, anchovies and black olives)
Handful raw pumpkin seeds

SNACK

10 raw, sprouted almonds (p. 65) with
1 glass kefir (cultured yogurt drink)
Flat Tummy Boost (p. 172)

DINNER

Sardine dip with gluten-free crackers (2
tinned sardines blended with 1 tbsp vegan
mayo, 2 tsp vinegar, 1 tsp mustard)
Feast: salad of tomatoes with basil,
cucumber, steamed asparagus, olive oil
and crushed garlic
Ginger tea

DAY 4

BREAKFAST

Juice of ½ lemon in 125ml
room-temperature water
1 cup peppermint tea
2 slices gluten-free, yeast-free bread
1 mashed avocado with fleur de col or Maldon
sea salt and pinch cayenne pepper (optional)
1 handful raw almonds

LUNCH

Steamed artichoke with Yogurt Sauce (p. 80),
plus pinch cayenne pepper
Swede purée with grilled wild salmon

SNACK

Buckwheat Crêpe (p. 71)
1 tbsp homemade Almond Butter (p. 225)
Cinnamon tea

DINNER

Feast: stir-fried Brussels sprouts, cabbage
and kale (shred and sauté briefly in olive oil;
add crushed garlic and lemon juice)
Grilled turkey breast
Cream of Chia Seed and Coconut (p. 170)
Ginger tea

DAY 5

BREAKFAST

Juice of ½ lemon in 125ml room-temperature water
1 cup peppermint tea
Gluten-free granola (mix of almonds, sunflower seeds, pecan nuts, coconut and cinnamon), served with 250ml coconut milk with vanilla extract

LUNCH

Salad of wild tuna, wheat-free pasta and olives
Tomatoes and grated courgette with Lemon Vinaigrette (p. 83)

SNACK

10 raw, sprouted almonds (p. 65) with 1 glass kefir (cultured yogurt drink)
Cinnamon tea

DINNER

Tortilla Soup (p. 168)
1 handful raw almonds
Raw Chia Seed Pudding (p. 172)
Ginger tea

DAY 6

BREAKFAST

Juice of ½ lemon in 125ml room-temperature water
1 cup peppermint tea
Cinnamon Buckwheat Cream (p. 167)

LUNCH

2 herring fillets (tinned)
Italian Aubergines (p. 169)
10 raw, sprouted almonds (p. 65) with 1 glass kefir (cultured yogurt drink)

SNACK

1 Buckwheat Crêpe (p. 71)
1 tbsp homemade Almond Butter (p. 225)
Cinnamon tea

DINNER

Mock Mash (p. 238)
Salad of baby spinach leaves with Lemon Vinaigrette (p. 83)
Ginger tea

DAY 7

BREAKFAST	Juice of ½ lemon in 125ml room-temperature water 1 cup peppermint tea 2 Buckwheat Crêpes (p. 71)
LUNCH	Wild Salmon and Fennel Purse (p. 169) **Feast:** seasonal berries
SNACK	10 raw, sprouted almonds with 1 glass kefir (cultured yogurt drink) Cinnamon tea
DINNER	Gluten-free crackers Hummus (p. 70) Guacamole (p. 170) Tomato, cucumber, asparagus and walnut salad with Garlic Vinaigrette (p. 82) 4 tbsp homemade apple purée (p. 64) Ginger tea

BOOSTER
RECIPES

CINNAMON BUCKWHEAT CREAM

Serves 2
Preparation 5 min

Ingredients
150g sprouted (or not) buckwheat
120ml Almond Milk (p. 137)
1 tbsp hemp seeds
1 tbsp ground cinnamon
3 tbsp grated coconut

This healthy breakfast dish is a great way to kick-start the day.

1   Put all the ingredients in a blender.

2   Blend until smooth. Transfer to bowls and serve immediately.

LINSEED PORRIDGE

Serves 1
Preparation 10 min, plus soaking time

Ingredients
50g buckwheat seeds, soaked for 12 hours (or overnight) in 250ml filtered or still mineral water
100ml Almond Milk (p. 137), plus a little extra (optional)
2 tsp agave syrup
1 tsp linseeds
2 drops orange essence
a few almonds

Linseeds or flax seeds are an amazing source of omega-3 fatty acids, antioxidants, minerals and essential vitamins. I like to sprinkle these power seeds over my dishes as often as possible. You can use lemon or vanilla essence, if you prefer, in place of the orange essence.

1   Drain and rinse the buckwheat seeds thoroughly to wash off the gelatinous liquid.

2   Put the buckwheat, almond milk, agave syrup, linseeds and orange essence in a blender and mix until smooth.

3   Let the porridge rest for a few minutes and add more almond milk, if necessary.

4   Transfer to bowls and top with almonds, to serve.

TORTILLA SOUP

Serves 3
Preparation 15 min

Ingredients

½ onion, chopped
2-4 cloves garlic, crushed
1 tbsp olive oil
1 tsp cumin and 1 tsp cayenne pepper (optional)
1 x 400g tin chopped tomatoes
150g leftover cooked chicken
1-2 spring onions, chopped
about 2 tbsp chopped, fresh coriander leaves (discard the stems)
80g sweetcorn (tinned or frozen; optional)
1 litre chicken stock (fresh or stock cube), heated
salt and freshly ground black pepper, to taste
organic corn tortilla chips (check the label carefully), crushed

This is the fast-track version of a classic recipe. To fully develop the flavours, I suggest you leave it to simmer gently for one hour over a low heat. When you're not following the BOOSTER phase and avoiding yeast, you can adapt this by adding 1 tsp cumin and 1 tsp cayenne pepper for a subtle kick. If you use a stock cube, choose one that is low in sodium and contains no MSG.

1   Sauté the onion and garlic in olive oil until softened (if you are using cumin and cayenne pepper, add them now).

2   Drain the tomatoes, reserving the juice in case you need to add more liquid later. Add the tomatoes to the pan, together with the chicken, spring onions, coriander and sweetcorn, if using. Mix together.

3   Add the heated chicken stock and chopped tomatoes and heat through gently.

4   Season with salt and pepper, to taste. Be sparing with the salt if you've used a stock cube. Ladle into bowls and sprinkle the crushed tortillas over the top.

ITALIAN AUBERGINES

This dish is very satisfying by itself or with a side salad.

Serves 1
Preparation 40 min

Ingredients
1 tbsp olive oil
1 medium aubergine, peeled and diced
1 garlic clove (or more, if you like), crushed
450ml sugar-free tomato passata
½ tsp herbes de Provence, or herbs of your choice (I don't really measure)
sea salt, to taste
140g chickpeas or black beans

1   Heat the olive oil in a large frying pan over a medium heat.

2   Add the diced aubergine and sear for a few minutes, adding the garlic at the last minute.

3   Meanwhile, mix the passata, herbs, salt and beans in a bowl.

4   When the aubergine is done, place in an ovenproof dish and pour the tomato mixture over the top, coating it with the sauce.

5   Cover and bake at 180°C/350°F/gas mark 4 for 25–30 minutes.

WILD SALMON AND FENNEL PURSE

Fennel is an amazingly powerful detoxifying food and salmon is a fantastic source of healthy fats and good protein.

Serves 1
Preparation 30 min

Ingredients
1 Buckwheat Crêpe (p. 71)
1 wild salmon steak
1 large fennel bulb
1 tbsp olive oil
pinch of Fleur de Sel (or Maldon salt)
¼ tsp cayenne pepper
½ lemon, to serve
a few sprigs chives, finely chopped

1   Make the crêpe, place on a warmed serving plate, cover with foil and keep warm.

2   Steam or sauté the salmon to your liking.

3   Slice the fennel thinly, then cook gently in the oil until transparent and turning golden.

4   Scatter the fennel over the crêpe. Place the salmon on the fennel and season with salt and cayenne pepper.

5   Squeeze over some lemon juice and sprinkle over the chives. Make a 'purse' by bringing the edges of the tortilla together and tying in place with kitchen string.

GUACAMOLE

Serves 2
Preparation 10 min,
plus 1 hour

Ingredients
2 ripe avocados
juice of 1 lime,
or to taste
½ onion
½ tomato
10 fresh
coriander leaves,
finely chopped
salt
cayenne pepper or
fresh chilli, finely
chopped (optional)

1   Cut the avocados in half and scoop
out the flesh. Keep the stones. Mash the
flesh with a fork and add fresh lime juice
to taste.

2   Finely chop the onion and tomato.
If you have the time, deseed the tomato.

3   Mix the ingredients by hand – never with
a blender or food processor – until roughly
combined and a chunky texture. Each
individual ingredient should still be visible.

4   Add the chopped coriander and salt,
to taste. If you like, add cayenne pepper
or fresh chilli.

5   Place the stones in the guacamole to
prevent it from going brown. Cover and
refrigerate for 1 hour before serving,

CREAM OF CHIA
SEED AND COCONUT

Serves 1
Preparation 5 min,
plus 1-2 hours

Ingredients
2 tbsp chia seeds
150ml low-fat
coconut milk
2 tbsp grated
coconut
1 tsp agave nectar
½ tsp vanilla extract
ground cinnamon,
to serve

This rich, creamy drink is refreshing as a
snack, delicious after a meal and perfect for
breakfast on the go. The coconut milk should
be low fat; even better if it's fresh, rather
than from a tin!

1   Put all the ingredients in a blender
and mix.

2   Leave in the fridge for 1-2 hours.

3   Enjoy with a sprinkling of ground
cinnamon.

PARISIAN CRUMBLE

Serves 4-6
Preparation 1 hour

Ingredients
(for a 20 x 30cm
ovenproof dish)
3 tbsp gluten-free
flour or cornflour
(maizena) (optional)
6 to 8 cups of mixed
berries, fresh or
frozen pineapple (or
any other fruit that's
in your kitchen!)
3 tbsp muscovado
sugar (optional)

*My gluten-free
crumble topping*
150g gluten-free
oat flour (or any
other gluten-free
flour: rice, flour mix,
quinoa)
50g buckwheat flour
100g almond flour
50g crushed flax
seeds
50g oat flakes
4 tbsp brown sugar
grated zest of 1
organic orange
½ tsp nutmeg
¼ tsp sea salt
6–8 tbsp non-
hydrogenated
margarine

Here is a healthy and yummy recipe that you can enjoy during your BOOSTER phase – and also throughout the rest of the programme. It's a vegan dish which uses non-hydrogenated margarine, and has a gluten-free, homemade crumble topping. This can be served as a dessert for a family meal, but because it has a low-sugar content, you could also enjoy it as part of your breakfast. You can use a large cup to measure the berries – you'll need around 400g fruit in total. Even if you don't follow the fruit quantities to the letter, it will still taste amazing. Enjoy by itself or with a homemade vanilla ice-cream (raw or vegan, of course!).

1   Preheat the oven to 180°C/350°F/gas mark 4.

2   In a large bowl, mix together all the ingredients for the crumble topping, apart from the margarine.

3   Add the margarine and mix into the crumble by hand using the tips of your fingers, until it resembles breadcrumbs. You now have a ready-to-use crumble topping.

4   If using very juicy fruits, mix the gluten-free flour or cornflour with the fruit and scatter the mixture evenly over the base of the oven dish (there's no need to put any oil, butter or flour in the pan first). Omit the flour or cornflour if the fruit is drier.

5   Cover the fruit with the crumble topping and add the sugar, if liked, to deepen the golden colour of this dish.

6   Bake in the oven for 35-40 minutes, until the fruit 'bubbles' (to use the expression of a little boy who saw me make this recipe!).

7   Remove from the oven. Leave to cool for 15 minutes.

FLAT TUMMY BOOST

Serves 1
Preparation 5 min

Ingredients
180ml Almond Milk (p. 137)
2 sprigs fresh mint
3 ice cubes
1 pinch matcha green tea powder
1 packet stevia or 1 tsp agave nectar

Fresh mint has been used for hundreds of years in North Africa and Southern European for its digestive properties. This boost is a great way to support your digestion and alleviate bloating.

1   Combine all the ingredients in your blender and whizz together.

2   Drink immediately!

RAW CHIA SEED PUDDING

Serves 4
Preparation 15 min, plus 2 hours

Ingredients
125g cashew nuts
250ml water
3 tbsp honey
1 tsp ground cinnamon
¼ tsp ground nutmeg
¼ tsp ground ginger
1 tsp vanilla extract, or 1 vanilla pod
¼ tsp sea salt
100g chia seeds

There are many different types of honey you can try here, but make sure it's always raw and organic. Chia seeds can be found in all wholefood stores. It's not mandatory to use a vanilla pod, but the flavour will be better! If you do use a pod, split it and scrape the seeds into the blender with the other ingredients. I use a Vitamix blender. This keeps for four days, covered, in the fridge.

1   Place all ingredients, except for the chia seeds, in a blender and blend to a creamy consistency. (Do not put the seeds in the blender or they will turn to mush).

2   Place the chia seeds in a serving bowl and pour the creamy mixture over them, stirring them in with a fork.

3   Cover and leave to stand for 2 hours (not in the fridge). Spoon into individual ramekins and serve at room temperature.

CHICKPEA PIE CRUST

Serves 4
Preparation 10 min

Ingredients
40g chickpea flour
20g organic oat bran
pinch of salt
1 probiotic yogurt (vegan)
1 large tbsp olive oil

You can use this for just about any savoury or sweet recipe where the pastry needs to be blind baked before adding the filling or topping.

1   Sift the flour into a large bowl.

2   Mix in the oat bran and salt, then gently add the yogurt, stirring it in with a spatula.

3   Drizzle in the olive oil until the dough forms a ball. Tip the bowl from side to side, using a circular motion. As you drizzle the oil in, the ball will form itself.

4   Refrigerate for at least 1 hour.

5   Take 2 silicone sheets or 2 sheets of greaseproof paper (this is ESSENTIAL as the dough will be soft) and place the dough between them.

6   Roll the dough out between the two sheets with a rolling pin.

7   Transfer to the fridge and chill for 15-30 minutes. Preheat the oven to 200°C/400°F/ gas mark 6.

8   Remove the top silicone or greaseproof sheet and place on a baking tray. If lining a pie dish, carefully remove both sheets first. Bake for 25 minutes.

9   Add the toppings or filling and return to the oven for 5-10 minutes.

MAINTENANCE

GOALS

Stabilise your weight
for ever

Lose the last few
pounds that remain

MAINTENANCE

FACT

- An obese or overweight body is acidic. A healthy and lean body is alkaline or neutral.

Rules of the MAINTENANCE phase

- We do one TD Day per week.
- We drink Sobacha every morning.
- We drink lemon juice with water every morning.
- We pay attention to our body pH and regulate it by following a healthy diet and choosing the right balance of alkalising and acidic foods.
- We follow the MAINTENANCE fitness plans, according to our level of fitness, moving up as we progress and squeezing in 25th-hour exercises whenever we can. We continue to challenge the body, never resting on our laurels.
- We manage our stress with abdominal breathing exercises.

We are now all set to start the last phase. Look at all the progress you have made since we first started on this journey together! You have educated yourself in nutrition and fitness. You now know the difference between the Glycaemic Index and the Glycaemic Load. You know how to enjoy your food without gaining a gram. You have put a winning daily routine in place. All credit to you for your perseverance and your amazing motivation.

Since you are moving onto the MAINTENANCE phase, it means you have lost 75 per cent of the weight you wanted to shed, as we can only stabilise and maintain your success once that is achieved. So, hats off!

Take your time!

If you launch into MAINTENANCE too early, you can say goodbye to your achievements because you won't have waited long enough to 'stabilise' your new body. Undertake MAINTENANCE too late and your motivation might go down the drain. Timing is of the essence.

Let's refresh our memory. If you have reached a plateau during ATTACK, be patient and observe your benchmarking intervals – in other words, adjust your thinking so that your plateau weight is your new 'heaviest weight' each time. Remember to include a weekly TD Day and you will hit your target, guaranteed! You can also add an extra 30-minute walk per day and, most importantly, make sure you regularly document what you are doing in your blog to identify better your 'diet saboteurs', as I call them.

Check again that you are not repeatedly falling for a rich afternoon snack with your colleagues. Remember, two slices of cake means that more than 800 calories sneak into your diet. And you must know by now that 7,000 calories is all it takes to gain 1kg of fat!

Have you followed my plan to the letter? Have you jumped directly from a plateau in ATTACK, to MAINTENANCE, without completing your BOOSTER? Do you take your morning lemon juice? Do you drink your Sobacha? In short, question yourself honestly, and very quickly you will find the culprits, eliminate them and get back on the right track.

If you haven't lost 75 per cent of the weight you'd like to shed, I compel you to kick-start your weight loss with a BOOSTER, before returning to ATTACK. Only move onto the MAINTENANCE phase once you've lost the 75 per cent!

MAINTENANCE FOR LIFE

If you've succeeded and reached your 75 per cent goal, then bravo!
Now let's get started with the MAINTENANCE phase.

What is the point in stabilising your new weight? After all we have
already spent several weeks (or months) together, and you are lighter
and full of energy. You might think that we could perfectly well stop
right away and enjoy our new body.

I am the first one to acknowledge that it is very tempting to tell
ourselves all is going well, the goal has been reached and that we
can manage on our own. However, if the vast majority of dieting
attempts are met with failure – where we regain all the weight lost
or, worse, gain even more – it is very often because we don't take the
time to underpin our weight loss. (Not to mention the fact that some
diets are dangerous or simply ineffective.)

On the basis of evidence from numerous studies, I have designed
LeBootCamp Diet to include a MAINTENANCE phase that lasts at least
as long as your ATTACK phase, and which you then adopt permanently
so that it becomes part of your new life.

Why so long? Simply for you get to used to your new body, so that
it becomes the permanent 'new you', and so that you're never, ever
tempted to go back to your 'before' body. The only way to achieve this
is to learn how to maintain.

This phase will also serve to identify small problems that you might
still face. (That's why I say that MAINTENANCE is the phase where
you are going to lose the remaining 25 per cent.)

WHY SHOULD WE LEARN HOW TO MAINTAIN?

The importance of learning how to maintain has been proven beyond
any doubt. A large-scale study by researchers from Penn State
University (published in *The American Journal of Preventive Medicine*)
concluded that regaining weight after a diet is not inevitable, since we
now know how to stabilise weight indefinitely.

Most significantly, the study also revealed that the methods required to keep weight off are *not* the same as the ones used to lose weight in the first place. According to the author of this study, Dr Christopher Sciamanna (Professor of Medical and Public Health Sciences at Penn State College of Medicine), "Losing weight then stabilising one's new weight shares similarities with love and marriage. The reasons that take you to the altar are different from those which keep you married in the long run".

The researchers interviewed over 1,100 people who had lost and never regained a significant amount of weight. From these interviews, they identified 36 techniques for weight loss and maintenance. They then conducted a large national poll asking people who started with a BMI of greater than 25 (i.e., overweight) to confirm which of those 36 techniques were the absolute best ones.

One of the key findings was that successful dieters had followed a *clearly identified weight-loss programme* (as opposed to little tips gleaned here and there) – like LeBootCamp Diet, for instance! They had also reduced their sugar consumption, had not skipped any meals and kept fit following a philosophy of Easy Fitness.

The study showed that the four most successful strategies for stabilising the new weight (not necessarily valid in the weight-loss phase) were:

1   Adopt a diet with an adequate protein intake (vegetable or animal).
2   Follow a simple but consistent fitness routine.
3   Reward yourself (sensibly) each time you reach a milestone.
4   Regularly remind yourself of the reasons why you don't want to regain the lost weight.

Does this sound familiar? That's because these points echo the fundamental principles of LeBootCamp Diet. That is why you can trust me when I say that my method truly works: it has been scientifically proven to do so!

As we've just seen, we need the MAINTENANCE phase because the techniques needed to stabilise weight are different from those we used to lose it. I am asking you to follow this phase faithfully. Your success depends upon your commitment to the programme. So, keep up the great work. We are not quite done yet!

The conclusion of Dr Sciamanna's study, which is a key reference in the weight-loss world, is that the main difference between dieters who remain slim their entire life and those who fall continually into the vicious circle of losing, then regaining weight, is their state of mind and their level of motivation.

That is why the fourth concept we are going to explore together, central to the MAINTENANCE phase, is the concept of body pH. Why? Simply because not only does an acidic body make it harder to lose weight, but an acidic body is a tired body, without energy or stamina, which in turn affects our motivation level. A poor pH balance also triggers a slowdown in metabolism. As we know, a healthy metabolism is one of the cornerstones of weight loss and its maintenance. So – we need to work on our pH to support healthy weight loss. Simple!

In the DETOX phase we introduced the concept of detoxification; in the ATTACK phase, we learned how properly managing the glycaemic load of a meal can help limit insulin peaks, which transform us into fat-storing machines. In the BOOSTER phase, we learned about the connection between yeast and a flat stomach. Now, in the MAINTENANCE phase, we will discover how handling our body pH correctly can help us stay on the path of healthy and permanent weight loss.

(In fact, since you began this programme, you have been rustling up alkalising menus and recipes without realising it!)

What constitutes 70 per cent of our body, is pure, has a neutral taste and a perfect pH? WATER! And that's what our pH should be, as well. Throughout my programme we are working hard to come as close as possible to this ideal number. You will see how easy it is shortly.

In chemistry, the pH is a measure of the acidity or basicity of a solution. If the pH is less than seven then we say it is acidic and if it is greater than seven we call it basic or alkaline. Pure water has a pH very close to seven, which we also call neutral pH.

Why is seven a neutral value? Just as we've seen for the glycaemic index in ATTACK, the pH calculation is based on a reference value: that of pure water at 25°C.

pH VALUE	LEVEL
0–6.9	Acidic
7	Neutral
7.1–14	Alkaline

Although the pH of any solution can go from zero to 14, when it comes to our body the range is from five to nine with an average at 7.35 (for the urine pH). Although you can measure the pH of blood, organs, saliva and skin, please note that we will stick to measuring urine. Why? Because it is a very easy and painless procedure and a pretty accurate way to get a good reading of the state of our body.

The urine pH of a healthy individual who feeds herself correctly will be between 6.5 and 7.5. Just to illustrate my theory, here are two extreme examples:

- A sedentary, obese person who eats exclusively processed foods and red meat will have a pH inferior to seven and close to five – so, very acidic.
- A slim, healthy and active person who eats a balanced diet, with wholefoods, will likely have a pH close to seven (neutral).

Our body needs to be at a stable pH level simply for us to stay alive! Indeed, the value of our pH conditions a large number of chemical and enzymatic reactions which allow our cells to fulfil their functions. The closer our pH is to seven, the better our organs can function. The body does not need to consume energy to regulate its acidity level and can focus on other problems. Numerous studies have shown that an optimal pH level equips the body to prevent certain illnesses and sometimes even fight them. This seems to be the case, according to some studies, for cancer, osteoporosis, some allergies, arthritis and rheumatism.

When all is balanced, we feel better in our body, hence in our head, and we're at the peak of our vitality. Our resulting improved digestion contributes to a stable weight.

On the other hand, an acidic pH leads to the accumulation of acids in the tissues, causing inflammations, demineralisation and high blood pressure. In turn, those conditions can lead to osteoporosis, rheumatism, cancer, kidney disease (since the kidneys have to work double-time to compensate for excess acidity), diabetes and obesity.

Sadly, this list is not exhaustive since even a small pH fluctuation can lead to a multitude of consequences.

How and when should you measure your body pH?
It's very easy. You can measure it first thing in the morning by using pH strips (these are available at any chemist).

To be in the healthy range the pH of your first morning urine should be at 6.5 and above. Since this pH has not been affected by any drinks, foods, stress and so on, I like to call it your basal pH. If you are already at 7.3 you are doing GREAT and your basal level is simply perfect. Now you will need to make sure you don't bring it lower throughout the day by letting stress take over or by eating poorly.

If your basal pH is too low (under 6.5), you are acidic. This means you need to raise it by doing the right things: drinking alkalising fluids, eating well, and managing stress as much as possible, to bring your pH closer to seven or even better, above. (It's better to be slightly alkaline, because the body can easily become acidic, so this gives us more margin for staying the right side of neutral).

Ideally I would like you to test your pH every day, starting tomorrow: in the morning (and if, like me, you like to go the extra mile, during the day and at night). By doing this you will have a clear understanding of whether you have a healthy basal pH, made acidic by the way you lead your life, or, if you have a not-so-good pH at the start of your day, which you are able to change to neutral or alkaline by doing the right things.

It is also very possible that your morning pH is perfect and that it stays that way. Indeed, we have spent a few weeks together already, so if you have followed my programme to the letter, it is very likely that your pH is at a healthy level. If this is the case let's stay on the right track!

> **NOTE** In order to keep track of your pH evolution I suggest you record it in the blog you have been keeping during our journey together.

Why can't my healthy body take care of its own pH?
This is a question that I hear very often, both from journalists and BootCampers. Let's look first at how the body regulates pH. Two major organs support body pH balancing: our lungs and our kidneys.

Lungs: if your body becomes too acidic (with a low pH) it will respond by hyperventilating. It transforms the ions responsible for the acidosis into carbon-dioxide (CO_2) and steam. When carbon-dioxide levels in the blood are too high, the lungs start hyperventilating in order to exhale the CO_2, thus regulating its pH.

Kidneys: when hyperventilation is not enough to eliminate excess CO_2, our kidneys take over and expel hydrogen ions into the urine, in the form of ammonia. This is what turns your urine acidic. If acid levels become toxic, the kidneys are able to raise pH levels by reabsorbing bicarbonate ions.

It seems that our body is well equipped to face any pH challenge. However, the way we live today – high levels of oxidative stress, a poor diet and a sedentary lifestyle – can turn our pH levels chronically acidic. So, we need to support our body in order to maintain the correct pH level in the same way that our detoxifying functions also need support at pH level.

HOW TO BOOST YOUR pH

1   The problem: LACK OF OXYGEN

As we've just seen, the body uses breathing as a defence mechanism for balancing acidity levels. But do we truly take the time to breathe correctly and get as much oxygen into our body as we need? We lead increasingly sedentary lifestyles and are constantly exposed to pollution. We live in houses and office spaces that are over-heated, over-air-conditioned or poorly ventilated. This leads to a lack of oxygen in our system, which in turn leads to an increase of carbon-dioxide in our blood. The result? Our body cannot ventilate itself properly, and is thus unable to eliminate acid effectively.

Increased stress levels have also been strongly linked to a lack of oxygen, since a stressed person may have a tendency to slouch, thereby compressing the thorax and diminishing lung capacity. You must have noticed it: when you are under pressure your breathing is so shallow that very soon you need to take a deep breath. This is concrete evidence that you don't have enough oxygen in your body.

The solution: GET YOUR OXYGEN FIX

Getting the right amount of oxygen into your body will have a hugely positive effect on your pH. Use these simple techniques to clear acidosis and reduce the feeling of tiredness:

Ventilate! Health professionals advise us to change the air in our house for at least 10 minutes per day to eliminate dust mites and other micro-organisms in our mattresses. This also replaces some of the carbon-dioxide you generate during the night, with oxygen. Change the air at least every morning in each room of your house and once more in the afternoon if you work from home. Also, when you open the windows in the morning use this opportunity to do two minutes of intense abdominal breathing like we saw in the DETOX phase: inhale through both nostrils while inflating your abdomen as well as your thorax, then exhale through the mouth while sucking in your abdomen and emptying your lungs as much as possible.

Breathing fresh air is stimulating because it helps increase the level of oxygen in your body, thereby reducing the excess carbon-dioxide in your blood. If you want to see how powerful this technique is, stay in an unventilated office space all morning and you will see how exhausted you feel by lunchtime. Then, go out – jog, run, walk at a fast pace, taking care to inhale and exhale fully. Just 10 minutes are enough to witness a miracle: your energy is back! How impressive that only a 10-minute walk outside can restore your pH balance.

Move more! Beyond the regular physical activity one needs to perform in order to be healthy, make sure you get your daily walking fix. Remember my famous 30 minutes on an empty stomach? Keep it going and make it a habit for life!

Get taller! Adopt a good posture when you are sitting at your desk, driving, eating   even when you are walking. Stand tall and gently rotate your shoulders and neck; open your upper body by drawing your shoulder blades together. This posture will not only protect your back and help increase your lung capacity, but it will also send your self-confidence soaring.

Go green! Take advantage of the weekend to take your family and friends to a park or the countryside, far away from the city, or at least away from polluted areas and main roads. Just enjoy the moment: far removed from the noise (less stress), with purer air all around (better for your oxygen levels).

Go even greener! It's a fact: some plants are not only a great help in reducing the level of pollution in your house but can also purify the air you breathe. They capture carbon-dioxide during the day and produce oxygen. Though you might have heard that they produce CO_2 during the night, in fact, plants actually absorb more CO_2 than they make and produce more oxygen than they absorb.

So, place plants everywhere in your house. Studies by NASA Phyt'air programme and the Faculty of Pharmacy at the University of Lille, France, show that the spider plant (chlorophytum comosum) has undeniable purifying qualities. In 24 hours, the chlorophytum plant can absorb over 86 per cent of the formaldehyde and 96 per cent of the carbon-monoxide in the air of a closed, average-sized bedroom. It makes the air in our house more breathable and helps alleviate allergy symptoms.

2   The problem: STRESS

We know already that overwork, lack of sleep and stress slow the elimination of metabolic toxic waste (as well as causing a lack of oxygen in our system, see above). This has been proven to lower our body's pH, thereby inducing a state of acidosis.

The solution: MOVE TOWARDS A STRESS-FREE LIFE

Easier said than done, you might think. Though we do need to keep a certain level of positive stress, we also need to reduce negative (or oxidative) stress as much as possible since this speeds up our cells' ageing process and considerably reduces our body pH.

Here are a few tips to help you achieve this goal.

Move! We know that physical activity increases the oxygen in our system. It is also proven that if you move regularly, whether by walking around the block, playing a game of sports with friends or going to a group fitness class you can boost your morale and your energy levels. And if you consider the fact that you also burn calories in the process, you can kill two birds (or three, in this case) with one stone.

Breathe! Stress, exhaustion, pressure ... there are so many situations where a little respite is needed. Practice my breathing routines (or 'breathing yoga') regularly to help empty your mind and get energised (pages 41 and 44). They will help reduce pressure, increase your oxygen levels and bring a feeling of well-being (and hence a higher pH). Do these as soon as you feel you need them – better still, don't even wait for the point of no return; make breathing yoga a daily routine, just like brushing your teeth.

3   The problem: POOR DIGESTION

Again, our busy lifestyle is the culprit here. We work further and further
away from where we live. We cut our lunch break short to finish an
urgent project so that we may make it back home in good time. Eating
on the go is commonplace, as is eating at our desk – we don't even
take the time to sit in a separate area. Enjoying breakfast with the
entire family is an event so rare that we have to plan for it – a sad
reminder of what our mornings have become: a race against time.

Worse still, we don't bother chewing our food (and chewing is such a
critical part of the digestive process). Because we don't take the time
to eat properly, our ability to digest deteriorates. Poor digestion leads
to constipation (lovely!), bloating and gas as well as toxic waste that
our liver will have to work hard to eliminate. With all this going on, it's
no wonder our body has no energy left to regulate our pH levels!

The solution: TAKE TIME OVER MEALS
- Sit down for lunch: avoid eating on the run, in your car,
  or standing in your office or at your desk.
- Allow yourself 20 minutes *minimum* for lunch.
- Chew each bite five to seven times.
- Put down your fork between bites.

4   The problem: AN UNBALANCED DIET

The modern Western diet usually contains too many acidic foods
(too much animal protein, processed meals, ready meals and so on)
and not enough alkaline foods.

The way we preserve, cook and eat food can also have a negative effect
on our pH balance: the over-processing of grains; a drastic reduction
in our consumption of raw fruit and vegetables; too much sodium, too
many flavour enhancers, artificial colourings, texturisers, and so on.
All of these contribute to an acidosis that our body cannot regulate if
it becomes too frequent.

The solution: IMPROVE YOUR DIET, STEP BY STEP

This is certainly the most important factor towards improving your
pH, but any dietary changes should be done at your own pace. I don't
recommend radically altering all your eating habits because that is
the best way to feel discouraged by the mountain of things you need
to change. Take it one step at a time and you will win this battle!

MAINTENANCE FOOD GUIDE

FOOD CATEGORIES	ALKALISING FOODS To feast on	ACIDIFYING FOODS To limit
Vegetables and pulses	All green vegetables, raw or cooked (asparagus; cruciferous veg such as broccoli, cabbage, kale; lentils; cucumbers; green beans; peas; salad leaves); plus aubergines, carrots, celery, potatoes, sweet potatoes	Most pulses (apart from lentils) olives, sweetcorn, winter squash
Meat and fish		Fish (though wild Alaskan salmon is the least acidifying), seafood, all meats
Dairy and eggs	Raw, unpasteurised milk (preferably sheep's or goat's); homemade, plain yogurt; cottage cheese; eggs	All other dairy
Drinks	Sobacha (p. 71), green tea, water; LeBootCamp alkalising drinks (p. 222)	Coffee, black tea, alcohol, fizzy drinks

FOOD CATEGORIES	ALKALISING FOODS To feast on	ACIDIFYING FOODS To limit
Fruits	Practically all fruits: apples, bananas, dates, grapes, lemons, kiwis, melons, oranges, peaches, pears, pineapples, raspberries, strawberries, tomatoes	Blueberries, plums, prunes, tinned and glazed fruits
Nuts, seeds, grains and soy	Almonds, chestnuts, hazelnuts, millet, soy, tofu, flax seeds, sprouted seeds, sunflower seeds, pumpkin seeds	Brazil nuts, pecans, porridge oats, walnuts, all grains
Spices, seasonings	Apple-cider vinegar, cinnamon, curry powder, garlic, ginger, onions, herbs, miso, mustard, sea salt, tamari	Ketchup, pepper, white vinegar
Other foods	Stevia, xylitol, seaweeds, bee pollen	Bread, pastries, pasta, sugar, sucralose, corn syrup, carob, cocoa

Even though I recommend reducing acidifying foods to a minimum it is essential – critical, even – that we don't get carried away and demonise acidifying foods. Indeed, just because a food is acidifying does not make it a poison. In the same way as with the so-called 'good' and 'bad' cholesterols, what matters is to strike the right balance between alkalising and acidifying foods.

In a well-balanced diet one should never, ever exclude entire food groups. It's all about balance, and reducing the percentage of acidifying foods in our diet. This healthy strategy will help us stay on the right track without becoming obsessive about counting points, calories and grams; or depressed because we have to remove some of our favourite foods from our life.

For instance, wholegrain bread is acidifying. However, because it contains important ingredients that are good for us such as fibre, magnesium and vitamin B2, it should still be included in a healthy diet. Cereal products and high-protein foods, like meat and some cheeses are very acidic. That is the reason why people who follow a high-protein diet have an acidic body, acidic-smelling sweat and noxious breath. The adverse effects of such a diet on the kidney system have been demonstrated time and time again.

You may be surprised to see lemons in the list of alkalising foods. *Outside the body*, lemon juice is acidic (pH is below 7). Everyone knows this – it's a citrus fruit. *Inside the body,* however, when it has been fully metabolised and its minerals are in the bloodstream, its effect is alkalising, and it therefore raises the pH of the body. You will also notice that there are some acidifying foods which I ask you to limit, but which you are allowed to eat freely in the DETOX and ATTACK phase. Again, it's all about balance.

What is the ideal balance?
The ideal meal should consist of two-thirds alkalising foods and one-third acidifying foods. I am not asking you to constantly monitor what you are eating to reach the perfect balance.
This would become counter-productive and a source of anxiety (which we are trying to avoid!). Finding this balance will become easier after a few days of incorporating more and more alkalising foods into your diet.

Take the time to have a hard look at your plate, your friends' plates, even – and this is most revealing of all – other people's shopping trolleys at the supermarket checkout. You will realise that we usually do the opposite, with one-third alkalising foods and two-thirds acidifying.

Together, we are going to reverse this trend. The menus and recipes at the end of this chapter (page 220) are specially designed to help your body reach the correct pH balance.

Five steps to a healthy, alkaline diet

As well as aiming for the right balance of acidifying and alkalising foods, there are eating habits that you can adopt to improve your diet. Follow these guidelines *for life* and you'll also help to balance your pH.

1 Pass on the salt! As we know, salt is increasingly used in ready meals as a taste enhancer. It's far too easy to get too much of it, which can cause an acidic pH, cardiovascular problems, water retention, and so on. Limit your sodium consumption by cooking without salt and only adding it before serving or eating. Do not leave the salt shaker on the table – keep it far from the hand and far from the plate. Herbs, spices and other seasonings make ideal substitutes that will titillate your tastebuds without added calories, without sodium and, hence, without any impact on your health.

2 Go raw! How many raw vegetables did you tuck into last week? Include raw fruits and veg in your meals as often as you can. When I travel to France and to the UK, I often meet with BootCampers who tell me that uncooked vegetables make them feel bloated and give them an intolerable level of gas. This is most likely because they are consumed on an irregular basis. To avoid bloating, abdominal pain or cramping, it is critical to change your habits slowly. Just like a vegan would be afflicted by stomach pains should she switch to a meat-based diet overnight, a person who eats very few raw foods would suffer if her diet was changed abruptly.

Start with one serving a day, then two, then three, then more, at your own pace, so that your body has time to get used to this new way of eating.

If you did not eat raw foods at all before this programme, you will need about six weeks to get to the optimal level of raw food without suffering undue pain and bloating. If you were already eating some, you will need less time to adjust. I aim for eight servings a day of raw food: six of dark, leafy greens; or cruciferous; or sulphur-rich veggies like artichoke and asparagus, and two servings of berries or citruses.

3   Skip the processed food! Thanks to the food-manufacturing industry and its colossal marketing budgets we consume more and more refined products (ready meals, cakes, biscuits, fizzy drinks, white bread, white rice, pasta, and so on). But these foods and drinks have undergone so much processing that they have a negative impact on our body pH.

The vast majority of breakfast cereals contain so much sugar that they are actually unhealthy. A classic breakfast of orange juice from a carton, plus a bowl of cereal and milk (containing lactose, a sugar), represents a mega sugar-bomb right at the start of the day. Examine your choices: go for wholefoods, and alternate your glucids (bread, rice, pasta, buckwheat, quinoa) with pulses (lentils, chickpeas, edamame beans), all of which are richer in alkalising elements, fibre and minerals.

4   Eat your veggies! Our animal protein intake has greatly increased over the past few decades, replacing healthier vegan protein. This is clear when you think how we plan meals by choosing what will go with the meat or fish, rather than the other way round. Why not start by choosing first which vegetables and whole grains will make the base of your meal and only then decide if you need to add animal protein? If your meal already consists of vegetables or whole grains such as rice or buckwheat, then you can add tofu or pulses as a side dish to obtain the ideal vegan protein balance.

5   The right size! Remember what the size of a portion is, especially when it comes to animal protein (see DETOX, pages 59 and 60).

TOP 10 WAYS TO ALKALISE YOUR DIET

1 Lemon zest
Easy to add to your fruit salads and other homemade dishes. Go for organic, unwaxed citrus so you're not ingesting pesticides (remember, they are toxic for our body) and other chemicals.

2 Hazelnuts
You'll be familiar with my recipe for homemade Hazelnut Milk (p. 73) from the DETOX phase. The great news is that this nut is also wonderful for regulating your pH. Hazelnuts are rich in energy, so don't eat more than 15 for a snack with an apple, for example.

3 Avocado
Stay away from serving avocado with mayo – way too rich. Instead, enjoy half an avocado in a veggie sandwich or in a salmon tortilla (recipe on p. 84).

4 Fruit at every meal
You already start your day with fresh lemon juice. Now you can add a banana to your breakfast, make a colourful fruit salad for lunch and round off dinner with a berry crumble.

5 Veg: bring them centre-stage
Steamed artichokes with soy-based mayo; aubergines au gratin; steamed broccoli with a dash of olive oil and a pinch of sea salt; a red cabbage salad or mashed sweet potatoes – these are all easy-to-make dishes that will help you increase your pH, and don't have to be relegated to the side. Use the frozen versions to speed up the cooking process, any time of the year.

6 Sprouted seeds and grains
Sprouts are highly alkalising and becoming easier and easier to find. Simply top your salads with a few sprouts and, voilà! If you would rather make them yourself, here's a simple method. You don't need any dedicated equipment (though you might find seed-sprouters in health food stores or online). Begin with lentils, quinoa or alfalfa. Place the seeds or grains in a sieve above your kitchen sink. Each time you go through your kitchen, water them. After a few days (or a few hours, for quinoa) you will have the pleasure of seeing baby sprouts peeking out.

7 Onions, shallots, garlic and herbs
Commonly found all year round, these staples will spice up your meals while increasing your pH.

Bake a garlic head and serve it with roasted chicken or courgettes au gratin ... scrumptious! Add shallots to a vinaigrette and raise the culinary bar. Throw fragrant herbs into a simple salad and raise it to the next level. Add chives to a cauliflower purée; rosemary to a ratatouille; bay leaf to a potato gratin and your dishes will go from 'normal' to exotic and chic.

8   Soy and tofu

Replace dairy milk with plain soy milk in recipes that call for the real thing and you will be amazed at how delicious the dish tastes. Marinate cubed, firm tofu in equal parts of olive oil, reduced-sodium soy sauce, Dijon mustard and balsamic vinegar. Stir-fry them – and I guarantee your kids will love it. My teenage son always asks me, "When are you making your Dijon tofu again?" Edamame beans – like in Japanese restaurants – are also great as an appetiser.

9   Cinnamon and honey

Yum! A little bit of honey on a cubed apple over which you sprinkle some cinnamon; or a small coconut-milk yogurt with cinnamon – pure delight!

Choose organic honey and, if you can, also go local and raw (avoid honey heated to a very high temperature).

10 Potatoes and lentils

And you thought that to lose weight you had to banish potatoes from your diet? Not in the least!

Just like lemons, potatoes are acidic outside the body, but alkaline-forming when ingested (baked potatoes, with the skin, are the most alkaline-forming; even homemade chips are slightly alkaline. However, almost all commercial, fast-food chips are acidifying). They are also rich in potassium and calcium.

I am not saying you should tuck into them at every meal but if you love your roots then go for it: purple, blue, red. Try different types to discover new tastes and get the maximum amount of antioxidants (red or blue have the highest levels). Do the same with lentils and try beluga, coral, red, white or French lentils, in warm salads, Indian soups – the sky's the limit.

FITNESS TO STABILISE
YOUR WEIGHT LOSS

During ATTACK, we learned to diversify our exercise routine (you may have tried out zumba classes, aquabiking, tae bo, kickboxing, bokwa, pilates, yogalates and so on) because variety does wonders when one is trying to lose weight.

During the MAINTENANCE phase, however, you should find what works for you and stick to it. Studies have shown that you shouldn't be chopping and changing your exercise plan with something new every week. Now is the time to make choices, establish a regular routine you can enjoy and make it an integral part of your lifestyle. Of course there is no harm in trying out new sports or exercise classes once in a while, but not with the same butterfly attitude you might have done when you were in the ATTACK phase.

To maintain your new figure and even go a bit further, we are going to put in place a well-rounded fitness regime that will keep you motivated. Determine your fitness level (beginner, intermediate, or advanced) and commit to your exercise plan. It is so easy to find 'good' excuses not to work out: the kids need picking up from school; you have reached your perfect weight and can squeeze into your ideal clothes size; you are too busy with work; your boss has set a tight deadline for a new project; you're home too late or leave too early in the morning.

We women always seem to have too much on our plate (no pun intended) and neglect to place ourselves at the top of our priority list. To be able to love and take care of others, it's essential that you look after yourself. I assure you a good dose of personal TLC will go a long way. So, no more excuses. Carve out time for yourself. I know it might be annoying to be told, "If there's a will there's a way," but it's the truth! I do realise that this will be easier for some, but we can always find a way to do at least 'something'.

Four more 25ᵗʰ-hour exercises

My '25ᵗʰ-hour' exercises are easy, breezy routines that you can squeeze into a packed routine without even breaking a sweat. We have already learnt a few of them in DETOX (pages 46–49). Here are four new ones:

The Little Red Man
Waiting to cross the road? Don't waste this precious time! Standing straight, put all your weight on the right leg, bending the left one slightly and resting on the toes of your left foot. Discreetly push down your left heel while contracting your glutes. Repeat until it burns and then switch legs. If you don't have time to work the second leg, just do it at the next crossing!

The Moulin Rouge Secret to a Firm Derrière
A friend of mine who was a dancer at the famous Moulin Rouge cabaret in Paris shared this secret with me. Those ladies are required to display an exceptionally pert behind on stage. My friend told me that she never, ever, rested on her bottom without contracting it. Her theory is not scientifically proven (I state this clearly to avoid scrutiny from fitness professionals), but she claims that if we don't engage our glutes while we rest, we'll get a saggy bum – and we don't want that, do we?

Iron Adductors
Adductors are the muscles that run down the inner thighs, and you know how hard it is to tone them. I really dislike seeing my inner thighs flabby so I created this easy exercise which you can perform in bed. Lie on your back, arms along your body, legs straight and together. Open and close your legs as quickly as possible, pointing your toes. Put more thought in the 'closing' movement to really engage your adductors. Visualise squeezing a big balloon as you bring them together. Aim for 50 reps per day to get visible results after one month.

Strong Upper Arms
Hold a large (full) bottle of water in one hand, palm facing up, elbow tucked into your side, forearm straight ahead of you and parallel to the ground. Keep your back straight. Without moving your elbow, lower the bottle all the way down and raise it back up. Do not over-extend your arm, to avoid injuring your elbow. Repeat 20 times and change arms.

Three MAINTENANCE fitness plans

These plans are designed for three progressive levels: beginners, intermediate and advanced. If you are starting at the first level, do keep up with the pace. Move to the next programme once you feel the routine is no longer challenging you. You will shape yourself all the way up to advanced within a few months.

The one-hour walks can be taken during the day in chunks, if that's easier for you than walking the full extent in one go.

A selection of exercises follow the plans. You can vary the programme by swapping one exercise for another similar one from this book. For example, you could try *Gazelle Legs* (page 118) in place of *Leg Balancer*, but stick to the same duration for each day.

You should also keep fitting in as many 25th-hour exercises as possible.

To see me perform the exercises that follow go to www.lebootcamp. com/uk/exercises.

BEGINNERS

Monday	Butterfly Abs (50 reps); plus 30-min walk (ramble in the woods, the park, along the river or the beach); plus 5-min Metaboost #1.
Tuesday	30-min walk on empty stomach, steady pace; plus The Balancer (50 reps); plus 30-min walk; plus 5-min Metaboost #1.
Wednesday	30-min walk on empty stomach, steady pace; plus Butterfly Abs (50 reps); plus 30-min walk; plus 5-min Metaboost #1; plus 20 min of fitness exercises (such as zumba, body pump, strength-training, Doggy Paddle).
Thursday	30-min walk on empty stomach, steady pace; plus The Balancer (50 reps); plus 30-min walk; plus 5-min Metaboost #1.
Friday	30-min walk on empty stomach, steady pace; plus Butterfly Abs (50 reps); plus 30-min walk; plus 5-min Metaboost #1; plus 20 min of fitness exercises, as above.
Saturday	30-min walk on empty stomach, steady pace; plus The Balancer or Butterfly Abs (50 reps); plus 30-min walk (who said shopping wasn't a sport?); plus 1 cardio session (bike ride with friends, for example); plus 5-min Metaboost #1.
Sunday	30-min walk on an empty stomach, steady pace; plus The Balancer or Butterfly Abs (50 reps); plus 30-min walk; plus 5-min Metaboost #1; plus 30 min of fitness exercises, as above.

INTERMEDIATE

Monday

30-min brisk walk on empty stomach; plus Butterfly Abs (100 reps); plus 1-hour walk; plus The Balancer (100 reps); plus 20 min of toning exercises: Wall Press-ups, 45-degree Triceps, Leg Balancer, Doggy Paddle.

Tuesday

30-min brisk walk on empty stomach; plus The Balancer (100 reps); plus 1-hour walk; plus Butterfly Abs (100 reps); plus 10-min Metaboost #2.

Wednesday

30-min brisk walk on empty stomach; plus Butterfly Abs (100 reps); plus 1-hour walk; plus The Balancer (100 reps); plus 10-min Metaboost #2.

Thursday

30-min brisk walk on empty stomach; plus The Balancer (100 reps); plus 1-hour walk; plus Butterfly Abs (100 reps); plus 10-min Metaboost #2.

Friday

30-min brisk walk on empty stomach; plus Butterfly Abs (100 reps); plus 1-hour walk; plus The Balancer (100 reps); plus 10-min Metaboost #2.

Saturday

30-min brisk walk on empty stomach; plus Butterfly Abs or The Balancer (200 reps); plus 1-hour walk (window shopping counts); plus 1 cardio session (a long bike ride with the family, spinning class, running); plus 10-min Metaboost #2.

Sunday

30-min brisk walk on empty stomach; plus Butterfly Abs or The Balancer (200 reps); plus 1-hour walk (a hike in the woods, along the beach or the river); plus 20-min fitness session, with exercises of your choice.

ADVANCED

Monday	45-min brisk walk on empty stomach; plus Butterfly Abs (150 reps); plus Wall Press-ups (20 reps); plus 1-hour walk; plus The Balancer (100 reps); plus 20 min of fitness and toning (Wall Press-ups, 45-degree triceps, Leg Balancer, Vendetta Hammer).
Tuesday	45-min brisk walk on empty stomach; The Balancer (150 reps); Wall Press-ups (20 reps); plus 1-hour walk; plus Butterfly Abs (100 reps); 15-min Metaboost #3; 1 cardio session.
Wednesday	45-min brisk walk on empty stomach; plus Butterfly Abs (150 reps); plus Wall Press-ups (20 reps); plus 1-hour walk; plus The Balancer (100 reps); plus 20 min of fitness and toning (Reverse Triceps, Leg Balancer, Vendetta Hammer); plus 15-min Metaboost #3.
Thursday	45-min brisk walk on empty stomach; plus The Balancer (150 reps); plus Wall Press-ups (20 reps); plus 1-hour walk; plus Butterfly Abs (100 reps); plus 15-min Metaboost #3.
Friday	45 min brisk walk on empty stomach; plus Butterfly Abs (150 reps); plus Wall Press-ups (20 reps); plus 1-hour walk; plus 15-min Metaboost #4; plus The Balancer (100 reps); plus 1 cardio session (zumba or running).
Saturday	45-min brisk walk on empty stomach; plus The Balancer (250 reps); plus Wall Press-ups (20 reps); plus 1-hour walk (around the shops counts!); plus 1 cardio session (long bike ride with the family); plus 15-min Metaboost #3.
Sunday	45-min brisk walk on empty stomach; plus Butterfly Abs or The Balancer (250 reps); plus 1-hour walk (hike); plus 20-min fitness session with exercises of your choice.

ABDOMINALS

• Butterfly Abs
This exercise allows you to work your deep abs and get a flat and sexy tummy. Do this according to your programme – and, if you have time, increase to at least four times a week. More is good!

1   Sit comfortably on a gym mat or carpet with your legs in a diamond shape, with the soles of your feet touching. Don't worry if you aren't very flexible at the start. As you progress your knees will eventually reach the ground so that you create the perfect butterfly.
2   Place your hands under the nape of your neck. Inhale through your nose.
3   Raise your chest about 10cm while exhaling through your mouth (not forcefully).
4   Lower your chest to the starting position as you inhale, then exhale as you go back up again.
5   Repeat **25 times** and, as you progress, up to **50 times**. Yes, you can do it!

> **CAUTION** Do not push your head with your hands as this puts your neck at risk of injury. The purpose of your hands is only to keep your head in alignment with your back and shoulders. You don't want to curve your back like a turtle!

• The Balancer
For those who want a real challenge to tackle those deep abs, here is the absolute weapon. The Balancer is what we call a 'functional' exercise, because it uses the weight of the body (and a small nudge in the right direction with a medicine ball) to strengthen your muscles. You really have to keep your balance with this one!

You can do this anywhere: in your living room during ad breaks, in the morning after your walk, in the evening before going to sleep. You are the boss! I recommend you do this exercise once a day (which means going the extra mile, if your programme doesn't specify it). It takes two minutes and the results are visible almost immediately!

1 If you have fragile knees like me, I advise you to kneel on a gym mat, two beach towels, a carpet or rug.
2 Keep your back straight.
3 Take a medicine ball or full water bottle and hold it in front of you with arms slightly bent.
4 Keeping your stomach in, and your arms very slightly bent so as not to put pressure on the elbows, carry out a balancing move (a semi-circular motion, never reaching above your head): go from the right-hand side towards the left, moving upwards, and then return, moving downwards. A return round counts as 1 movement.

Beginners: 1kg weight; 3 series of 10 semi-circles; 15-sec rest between series.
Intermediate: 3kg weight; 3 series of 30 semi-circles; 15-sec rest between series.
Advanced: 6kg weight; 3 series of 50 semi-circles; 15-sec rest between series.

ARMS

Did you know that the shape of our arms can significantly impact how we perceive our body? Toned arms improve the overall body appearance of even a plumper person. As with your abs, toning up your arms doesn't require a superhuman effort or spending endless hours at the gym. You can work on your triceps and biceps throughout the day or in just a few minutes in the morning and at night.

Since the forearms are usually toned enough thanks to our daily activities, we won't need to focus on them.

• 45-degree Triceps
The triceps are located between your elbow and your shoulder on the back of your arm and are the hardest arm muscles to tone. This exercise is one I particularly love because it is quick, easy and incredibly efficient.

1 Take two weights (you can use two bottles or two tins of identical weight). Hold your weights in both hands and stand with your feet shoulder-width apart, abs tight.
2 Bend forward slightly at the waist, forming a 45-degree angle, starting from the waist. Inhale.

3   As you exhale, pull your arms back so that the upper part of your arms is in alignment with your torso, and your elbows are bent. This is the starting position.
4   As you inhale, push the weights back to straighten your arms and feel the contraction in your triceps.
5   Return your arms to the starting position as you exhale.

Beginners: 2kg weights; 3 series of 20 reps; 15-sec rest between series.
Intermediate: 4kg weights; 4 series of 25 reps; 15-sec rest between series.
Advanced: 6kg weights; 5 series of 30 reps; 15-sec rest between series.

> **TIPS** Be aware of your posture. Don't round or arch your back; keep it as straight as possible when you bend forward. Check your posture in a mirror if you can. Don't forget to breathe!

• Wall Press-ups

If you want to continue working your triceps, do 20 Wall Press-ups every time you go to the loo. We learned this one in DETOX, but here's a reminder:

1   Stand facing a wall, feet hip-distance apart, close enough to touch it with your arms straight out, at eye level.
2   Place your palms on the wall and bend at the elbows to do 20 standing press-ups.
3   Push your body back from the wall harder each time, moving slowly and maintaining control.

> **TIP** Increase the difficulty of this exercise by keeping your fingers off the wall, or by working only one arm at a time.

• Doggy Paddle

This exercise tones the deltoids – the muscles located at the tops of our arms towards our shoulders. Toned deltoids will make your upper body look fabulous in a sleeveless dress or bikini. You'll love wearing backless tops and spaghetti straps again!

This is my favourite way to work these muscles. Do this move whenever you hit the pool or beach!

1   Place flippers on your feet.
2   In the water, lie down on your tummy on a board or float.
3   Let your legs simply float on the surface of the water while your arms paddle.

> TIP You know this move is working when you feel the burn in your triceps, *not* your upper back.

• Reverse Triceps

You can do this at home using your sofa, your bed or a bath that's securely bolted in place; or in the park using a bench. After a few weeks you'll have toned, shapely arms and you'll be able to wear sexy, sleeveless dresses without feeling self-conscious.

1   Stand with your back facing the seat or support. Place your hands behind you on the seat, hip distance apart, and face forwards.
2   Walk your legs forwards until they are at a 90-degree angle. Keeping your back straight, use the force in your triceps to lower your body until your bum is just below knee level – do not let your body drop too far.
3   Slowly lift your body back up to its original position, controlling your triceps as you do so. Do not bounce. Try and maintain full control throughout.

Beginners: 2 series of 10 reps; 15-sec rest between series.
Intermediate: 2 series of 25 reps; 15-sec rest between series.
Advanced: 3 series of 50 reps; 15-sec rest between series.

• Vendetta Hammer
Do this exercise three times a week or according to your programme.
It will:

* Eliminate stress: simply visualise whatever it is that is causing you stress and pound it out. It really works!
* Tone your abs and 'core', namely the abdominal strap and lower back.
* Strengthen the muscles of your upper body and arms (anterior deltoids). I'll leave you to discover where else you feel the after-effects of the workout most on the following day!

1   Do this exercise **outside** so as not to hit anything, or in a room where you have enough space around yourself.
2   Take a heavy weight, according to your fitness level and strength, below; personally, a 10kg weight is enough for me for this exercise.
3   Standing with your legs shoulder-width apart, feet and toes pointing forward, knees slightly bent, back straight and abs contracted (yes, you can do it!), hold the weight in both hands.
4   'Launch' it above your head, maintaining control throughout. Don't throw the weight, but send it up in a controlled movement. **Hold on to the weight tightly** so that it doesn't slip out of your hands. It is also very important that your back and abs are nice and tight when you do this exercise, because if not, you can actually damage your back.
5   Return to the starting position by gently lowering the weight.

Beginners: 1kg weight; 1 series of 25 reps; 15-sec rest between series.
Intermediate: 5kg weight; 2 series of 25 reps; 15-sec rest between series.
Advanced: 12kg weight; 3 series of 30 reps; 15-sec rest between series.

• Leg Balancer

This exercise works your abductor and adductor muscles – inner and outer thighs – and will kill those saddlebags. I do this with a chair at home, or whenever I am in a park or anywhere with a bench. There's no need to be wearing any specific sports gear.

1 Stand straight and place your hands on the top of the chair or park bench.
2 Raise your right leg to the right side of your body, pointing your toes.
3 Slowly lower your leg and flex your foot, remaining in control of the movement and without swinging.
4 Don't rest your foot on the ground but continue the movement as you raise your leg up again on the same side.

Beginners. 2 series of 25 reps each side; 15-sec rests between series.
Intermediate: 2 series of 50 reps each side; 30-sec rest between series.
Advanced: 3 series of 100 reps each side; 30-sec rest between series.

> **TIP** For an added challenge, let go of the bench or chair that you were using to keep your balance!

Metaboosts

For those of us who are pressed for time, here is another way to squeeze in exercise every single day. Follow the Metaboost specified in the programme you are following (either Beginners, Intermediate, or Advanced) and always feel free to add extra ones into your day!

1   Metaboost 5 min (Beginners)

1-min march on the spot (warm up)
1-min squats (sit in the air – no chair! – with your knees bent at a 90-degree angle)
1-min Wall Press-ups (p. 204)
1-min Butterfly Abs (p. 202)
1-min march in place (cool down)
Or
1-min march on the spot (warm up)
1-min skipping rope
1-min Lunges (p. 116)
1-min side-to-side leaps over a broom on the floor
1-min march on the spot (cool down)
Or
5-min power walk around the block

2   Metaboost 10 min (Intermediate)

1-min march on the spot (warm up)
20 Jumping Jacks (p. 48)
20 side-to-side leaps
20 long jumps (jump in front of you as far as possible)
20 side jumps (this time, use a broom and jump over it from right to left and then left to right)
20 series of hopscotch (20 jumps on one leg, alternating legs)
1-min regular speed walk
1-min frog jumps
1-min power walk (using arms to pump)

1-min regular speed walk
1-min relaxed walk (cool down)
Or
10-min power walk around the block
Or
10 min on your stationary bike at home

3   Metaboost 15 min (Advanced)

1-min march on the spot (warm up)
20 Jumping Jacks (p. 48)
20 side-to-side leaps
1-min Wall Press-ups (p. 204)
1 min abs (of your choice)
1-min march on the spot
20 Jumping Jacks (p. 48)
20 side-to-side leaps
1-min abs (of your choice)
1-min squats (sit in the air   no chair! – with your knees bent
   at a 90-degree angle)
4 min POWER walk (1 min at normal speed, then 1 min at a
   very fast speed, and repeat)
2-min squats, while walking (walk, stop, squat; repeat)
1-min 'Sun Salutation Pose' (Stand on your mat. As you inhale,
   raise your arms over your head, keeping your palms together.
   Exhale and then slowly bend forwards, one vertebra at a time,
   until your hands touch your toes.)

MAINTENANCE
MENUS

To help you balance your body pH, I have put together two weeks of easy-to-follow menus with 14 alkalising recipes.

Should you struggle to produce some of the dishes or to find some of the ingredients I mention, just stick to those meals you enjoy preparing. You can repeat them as often as you like. For instance, if you only like one of my breakfast suggestions, then repeat it, as long as doing so is not boring (I like variety but some people prefer routine). In the end, you decide. This phase is more flexible than others, because MAINTENANCE is for life!

And don't forget, even during MAINTENANCE we stick to our weekly TD Day (page 97) to help keep our body as toxin-free as possible. By the same token, when you have gone overboard and indulged in too much rich food, insert a BOOSTER (page 152) to kick-start your weight loss.

DAY 1

BREAKFAST	Juice of ½ lemon in 125ml room-temperature water
	1 cup Sobacha (p. 71)
	2 Buckwheat Crêpes (p. 71) with Almond Butter (p. 225)
	Feast: blueberries or seasonal berries
LUNCH	Salad of ½ avocado, watercress, ½ pear and 1 tbsp Roquefort, with Mimosa Champagne Vinaigrette (p. 83)
	1 slice wholewheat bread with Hummus (p. 76)
	Feast: broccoli au gratin (cover steamed florets with 250ml milk mixed with 1 beaten egg, pinch nutmeg and 2 tbsp grated parmesan. Cook at 180°C/350°F/gas mark 4 for 10 min until browned)
	2 squares chocolate (your favourite) and 5 almonds
SNACK	1 glass Alkaline Lemonade (p. 221)
	1 apple, 3 dates and 15 hazelnuts
DINNER	**Feast:** cucumber salad with vinaigrette of your choice (pp. 82–83)
	Salmon steak en papillote (bake in lightly oiled parchment or foil, with lemon, seasoning, olives, tapenade, olive oil ... Use your imagination!)
	5 tbsp wholegrain rice
	1 soy yogurt

DAY 2

BREAKFAST
Juice of ½ lemon in 125ml
room-temperature water
1 cup Sobacha (p. 71)
2 Apple Buckwheat Pancakes (p. 224)
Feast: pink grapefruit

LUNCH
Feast: steamed asparagus with Balsamic
Vinaigrette (p. 82) or Soyannaise (p. 81)
Lentils with grilled chicken sausage
1 bowl raspberries

SNACK
1 gluten-free biscuit or slice of cake
(don't exceed 250 calories)
Feast: oranges

DINNER
Mock Mash (p. 238)
1 Vegetarian Burger (p. 237)
1 slice wholegrain rye bread
1 oven baked apple, sprinkled with
cinnamon

DAY 3

BREAKFAST
Juice of ½ lemon in 125ml
room-temperature water
1 cup Sobacha (p. 71)
1 Buckwheat Crêpe (p. 71) with a little
strawberry jam and a pea-size amount
of butter
1 Alkalising Boost (p. 221)

LUNCH
½ melon
1 small bowl Stir-fried Tofu with Dijon
Mustard (p. 78)
Baby potatoes sautéed in olive oil with garlic
Feast: 1 orange

SNACK
Raspberry and Coconut Smoothie (p. 223)

DINNER
2 slices proscuitto or serrano ham
Pondicherry Lentil Soup (p. 228)
1 plain soy yogurt with 1 tsp raw, organic
honey and a little cinnamon

DAY 4

BREAKFAST

Juice of ½ lemon in 125ml
room-temperature water
1 cup Sobacha (p. 71)
1 big slice toasted wholewheat bread
with cream cheese and 1 slice roast ham
Feast: seasonal fruit salad sprinkled
with cinnamon

LUNCH

Feast: Red Cabbage Gazpacho (p. 229)
Roast chicken breast (small portion)
Baked aubergine with Tomato Coulis
(p. 227)
1 banana

SNACK

1 cup green tea
Strawberry and Melon Soup (p. 242)
1 banana

DINNER

Salad of lamb's lettuce with seed sprouts
and Garlic Vinaigrette (p. 82)
Chilli con Carne (p. 240)
Fresh fruit salad, or whole fruit of your choice

DAY 5

BREAKFAST

Juice of ½ lemon in 125ml
room-temperature water
1 cup Sobacha (p. 71)
1 small bowl oat porridge (made with
coconut milk, cinnamon and 1 tsp raw,
organic honey)
1 Purple Boost (p. 222)

LUNCH

Vegetarian Burger (p. 237)
Sautéd Baby Broad Beans (p. 237)
1 slice wholewheat bread
Feast: kiwi

SNACK

1 Sweet and Mild Red Boost (p. 223), plus
Green-olive Tapenade (p. 227) on 1 slice
wholewheat toast

DINNER

Chicory salad with Garlic Vinaigrette (p. 82)
Trout en papillotte (see salmon, Day 1)
Feast: peas and carrots
1 soy yogurt and red berries

DAY 6

BREAKFAST	Juice of ½ lemon in 125ml room-temperature water
	1 cup Sobacha (p. 71)
	1 Buckwheat Crêpe (p. 71) with 1 tbsp Almond Butter (p. 225)
	Feast: papaya or pink grapefruit
LUNCH	Small bowl wholewheat pasta salad with a little feta cheese
	Feast: Spaghetti Squash with Mushrooms (p. 235)
	3 dried figs and 3 lychees
SNACK	Smoothie of banana and red berries, made with Hazelnut Milk (p. 73)
DINNER	Steamed leeks with Garlic Vinaigrette (p. 82)
	Escalope of turkey breast (bashed until thin and baked)
	Green beans with tomatoes (steam beans and sauté in 1 tbsp olive oil; add fresh, sliced tomatoes and oregano or basil)
	Feast: Pineapple Carpaccio (p. 241)

DAY 7

BREAKFAST	Juice of ½ lemon in 125ml room-temperature water
	1 cup Sobacha (p. 71)
	1 Buckwheat Crêpe (p. 71) with 1 tbsp Almond Butter (p. 225)
	1 bowl cottage cheese with apple and cinnamon
LUNCH	Grilled steak with caramelised onions (cooked in olive oil)
	Stir-fried veggies
	Soy yogurt and seasonal fruit
SNACK	Flat Tummy Boost (p. 172)
DINNER	**Feast:** Split-pea Soup (p. 230)
	2 slices wholewheat bread with Green-olive Tapenade (p. 227)
	1 peach and a handful raisins

DAY 8

BREAKFAST

Juice of ½ lemon in 125ml room-temperature water
1 cup Sobacha (p. 71)
1 Buckwheat Crêpe (p. 71)
3 tbsp unsweetened apple purée
1 pink grapefruit (see p. 88) or orange

LUNCH

2 slices gluten-free toast with Hummus (p. 76)
1 large, ripe tomato, sliced, with a drizzle of olive oil and basil
Feast: seasonal berries
4 squares chocolate (your choice)

SNACK

10 raw almonds
Feast: Papaya Granita (p. 241)

DINNER

Bok Choy with Prawns (p. 231)
1 banana

DAY 9

BREAKFAST

Juice of ½ lemon in 125ml room-temperature water
1 cup Sobacha (p. 71)
2 scrambled eggs cooked with 1 tbsp non-hydrogenated margarine
1 slice wholewheat toast
1 peach

LUNCH

Grilled fish of your choice with lemon wedges and 4 tbsp brown rice
Feast: steamed green beans
Small bowl fruit salad

SNACK

10 hazelnuts
5 tbsp homemade apple purée (p. 64)

DINNER

3 Beef Spring Rolls (p. 239) served with greens and fresh mint
Feast: seasonal berries

DAY 10

BREAKFAST

Juice of ½ lemon in 125ml
room-temperature water
1 cup Sobacha (p. 71)
Small bowl unsweetened muesli with
berries and 250ml vegan milk

LUNCH

1 small bowl kasha (roasted buckwheat
cooked in chicken or veg stock with
knife-end of butter or non-hydrogenated
margarine)
1 Vegetarian Burger (p. 237)
Feast: mandarins
1 coconut-milk yogurt

SNACK

10 walnuts
4 squares chocolate (your favourite)

DINNER

Chicory Boats with Smoked Salmon (p. 232)
Wholewheat pasta drizzled with olive oil
and 1 tbsp parmesan cheese
Feast: pink grapefruit (see p. 88) or orange

DAY 11

BREAKFAST

Juice of ½ lemon in 125ml
room-temperature water
1 cup Sobacha (p. 71)
Small bowl roasted buckwheat porridge
1 tbsp raw, organic honey
1 tsp raisins

LUNCH

Feast: minestrone soup (homemade,
or good-quality bought, with low salt)
1 slice honey-baked ham
1 small slice gluten-free toast
1 pear

SNACK

1 wholewheat pitta bread
3 tbsp Babaganush (p. 226)

DINNER

2 Vegetarian Burgers (p. 227)
Feast: salad of sliced cucumber with
white vinegar and dill
1 slice gluten-free toast
1 slice sheep's cheese
4 prunes

DAY 12

BREAKFAST

Juice of ½ lemon in 125ml
room-temperature water
1 cup Sobacha (p. 71)
1 Apple Buckwheat Pancake (p. 224)
2 tbsp Hummus (p. 76)
1 orange

LUNCH

Eat Out: 'Indian'
Vegetarian biryani
Palak paneer (spinach and paneer)
Feast: fruit salad

SNACK

10 raw almonds
1 banana

DINNER

Chicken Piccata (p. 238)
5 heaped tbsp steamed quinoa
4 squares chocolate (your favourite)

DAY 13

BREAKFAST

Juice of ½ lemon in 125ml
room-temperature water
1 cup Sobacha (p. 71)
1 plain croissant
Feast: orange

LUNCH

Dover sole en papillote (see salmon, Day 1)
Salad of steamed leeks with 1 tbsp Balsamic
Vinaigrette (p. 82)
1 slice goat's cheese
1 small slice wholewheat toast

SNACK

Feast: melon
10 walnuts

DINNER

Roasted Potatoes and Artichokes (p. 234)
1 Vegetarian Burger (p. 237)
4 squares chocolate (your favourite)

DAY 14

BREAKFAST	Juice of ½ lemon in 125ml room-temperature water
	1 cup Sobacha (p. 71)
	4 tbsp cottage cheese mixed with 1 tbsp honey, 3 tbsp unsweetened muesli and 1 peach
LUNCH	Veggie sandwich (raw or cooked, with wholewheat toast and 1 tbsp Soyannaise, p. 81)
	Feast: apple
SNACK	1 Flat Tummy Boost (p. 172)
DINNER	**Dinner with guests**
	Garden salad with Balsamic Vinaigrette (p. 82)
	Cabbage Blinis (p. 232) with roasted salmon fillets
	Poached Pears in Gooseberry Juice (p. 242)

MAINTENANCE
RECIPES

ALKALISING BOOST

Serves 1
Preparation 5 min

Ingredients
½ cucumber,
unpeeled
1 Asian pear,
unpeeled
2 slices ginger,
peeled

1 Place all the ingredients in your juicer.

2 Serve in a glass and enjoy right away.

ALKALINE LEMONADE

Serves 1
Preparation 5 min

Ingredients
juice of 1 ripe lemon
250ml semi-
sparkling water
10 drops stevia

This refreshing, naturally alkalising drink can be made in advance and consumed all day long. It will increase your body pH and keep your energy levels high. You can add colour by adding sprigs of mint, sliced strawberries, sliced cucumbers and so on. For a party, serve in a transparent water dispenser and add sliced oranges and sliced grapefruit.

1 Pour the fresh lemon juice into a glass and add the semi-sparkling water.

2 Add the stevia and mix well before tasting.

ALKALISING WATER

Serves 4
Preparation 5 min

Ingredients
½ cucumber
(unpeeled), sliced
½ lemon, sliced
1 litre water

Since lemon and cucumber are both highly alkalising, adding them to water will make a naturally alkalising drink. True, it's not as alkalising as fresh lemon juice but then this can cause thinning of tooth enamel if drunk all day long. If you're working from home, make this in a large jug. To take to the office, put the lemon and cucumber into a large water bottle and top up with water as the level goes down. The longer the cucumber and lemon stay in the water the more alkalising it is. If you're having a party, increase the quantities and serve this in a large water dispenser.

1   Place the sliced cucumber and lemon in a large jug.

2   Add fresh, cold water and leave for at least 30 minutes (at room temperature) before drinking.

PURPLE BOOST

Serves 2
Preparation 5 min

Ingredients
250ml Almond Milk
(p. 137)
100g blueberries
30g blackcurrants
1 banana
5 ice cubes
1 pinch cinnamon

This boost is a great morning pick-me-up that will super-charge your body with antioxidants and fibre. If you have a sweet tooth, then it's also a healthy way to satisfy your sugar cravings.

1   Put all the ingredients in the blender. Zap.

2   Serve immediately!

RASPBERRY AND COCONUT SMOOTHIE

Serves 1
Preparation 5 min

Ingredients
2 handfuls
raspberries
(preferably frozen)
½ tsp vanilla extract
1 tbsp Almond
Butter (fresh, if
possible; page 225)
250ml water
2 tbsp fresh,
grated coconut
(or dessicated)
1 tsp agave nectar
or raw, organic
honey (optional)

1   Place all the ingredients in a blender.

2   Pulse until well blended. Enjoy!

SWEET AND MILD RED BOOST

Serves 1
Preparation 5 min

Ingredients
1 apple
1 handful
strawberries
(fresh or frozen)
200g raspberries
(fresh or frozen)
1 orange, peeled

1   Rinse and pat dry the apple and strawberries and raspberries, if using fresh. Put them directly in the juicer with the orange. If you are using frozen fruit, juice the apple and orange first, transfer to a blender and add the frozen fruit (or it may damage your juicer).

2   Drink right away as antioxidants lose their potency as time passes.

APPLE BUCKWHEAT PANCAKES

Serves 2
Preparation 15 min

Ingredients
150g buckwheat flour
½ tbsp baking powder
½ tsp ground cinnamon
1 egg
4 tbsp homemade apple purée (p. 64)
250ml water
½ tsp vanilla extract
canola oil, for greasing, if necessary

This sweet buckwheat recipe can be used as a more indulgent (but still healthy!) alternative to the plain version in DETOX. It's great for breakfast, dessert or as a yummy snack after a long fitness session. Kids love it! I enjoy mine for my afternoon tea with a scoop of raw coconut ice-cream and fresh berries.

1   In a large bowl, combine the flour, baking powder and cinnamon. Mix well.

2   In a separate bowl, mix the egg, apple purée, water and vanilla extract. Add this to the dry mixture and stir until just combined.

3   Measure out about 1 small ladleful of batter onto a hot, non-stick pan or lightly oiled frying pan and cover with a lid, if your frying pan has one (this will keep the pancake moist).

4   Leave to cook over a medium heat until the centre starts to bubble and firm up.

5   Flip the pancake over and cook on the other side until golden brown.

6   Repeat the process until all the batter is used up.

GLUTEN-FREE PANCAKES

Serves 2
Preparation 15 min

Ingredients
50g chestnut flour, sifted
50g rice flour, sifted
2 tbsp ground almonds or hazelnuts
190ml rice or coconut milk
1 pinch salt
1 tsp canola oil

This is a great alternative for those with an allergy to Buckwheat Crepes (p. 71). Serve with agave syrup and fresh, seasonal fruit.

1   Mix all the ingredients, apart from the oil, in a large mixing bowl.

2   Heat a blini pan, or small frying pan, and add the oil.

3   Ladle small spoonfuls of batter into the pan to make blini-sized pancakes.

4   Cook over a medium heat for 2 to 3 minutes, flip and cook the other side until lightly golden.

ALMOND BUTTER

Serves 1
Preparation 5 min

Ingredients
2 handfuls raw almonds
2 tbsp orange juice or water (or 1 tbsp each)

I make this recipe at home all the time. You can also find almond butter in health food shops – some even make it fresh. It's a great alternative to regular butter, which contains a lot of saturated fats that are bad for our cardiovascular system. Use it in moderation!

1   Put the almonds with the 2 tbsp liquid in a powerful blender and whizz until you have a smooth paste.

2   Add a little more orange juice or water if the paste starts to clog the blender – but be careful not to add too much or the butter will be too runny.

BABAGANUSH

Serves 4
Preparation 40 min

Ingredients
3 medium
aubergines
juice of 1 lemon
5 anchovy fillets
(from a can, in olive
oil; optional)
2 tbsp mayonnaise
or Soyannaise (p. 81;
optional)
2 garlic cloves
80ml olive oil

Here is a great way to get your RDA of folic acid and potassium, both of which are found in aubergines and which are lacking in the typical Western diet. As much as I am opposed to using a microwave to cook because this type of heat destroys a lot of the antioxidants we are working on getting into our body, I use it here simply because it cuts the cooking time by two-thirds at least. Serve this chilled with pitta bread, Hummus (p. 76) and a few olives for a Middle-eastern combo plate.

1   Prick holes in the aubergines using a fork.

2   Cook them in the microwave on high for 8 minutes. Alternatively, place the aubergines on a baking dish, 2cm apart and bake for 20–30 min at 180°C/350°F/gas mark 4.

3   To check if the aubergines are ready, prick a few more holes in them. If your fork slides in easily then the aubergines are ready. They should also look a little 'deflated' when done properly.

4   Cut them in half and scrape the pulp into a food processor.

5   Add the lemon juice, anchovy fillets, mayonnaise or Soyannaise, 2 garlic cloves and olive oil.

6   Blend until smooth, or stop while you still have a coarse texture, if you prefer. I like mine completely smooth!

Variation: Add 1 tbsp tahini or 1 tsp ground cumin.

GREEN-OLIVE TAPENADE

Serves 2
Preparation 15 min

Ingredients
200g green
olives, pitted
2 anchovy fillets
1 tbsp capers
1 tbsp olive oil
freshly ground
black pepper

You can serve this tapenade on wholewheat toast, or shop-bought, good-quality parmesan cheese crackers. It's also delicious mixed with hot, wholewheat pasta for a quick lunch. It will keep for at least seven days in the fridge covered in clingfilm or a tight lid. I make mine in large batches which I keep and share with friends who come over. Nothing beats the sharing of home-made food!

1   Using a knife, coarsely chop the olives, anchovies and capers. Combine them in a bowl, then mash with a fork. Alternatively, for a coarser texture, whizz for a few seconds in a stand mixer or processor.

2   Add the olive oil and pepper.

3   Cover and refrigerate until ready to eat.

TOMATO COULIS

Serves 6-8
Preparation 45 min

Ingredients
2 x 400g tins whole,
peeled tomatoes
2 tbsp olive oil
1 tsp dried oregano
(or small bunch
fresh, leaves picked)
2 bay leaves (fresh
or dried)
2 garlic cloves
(1 crushed and 1
left whole)
2 thyme sprigs
salt and freshly
ground black pepper

You can play with the measurements in this easy, staple recipe and adjust them according to your taste. Make a batch ahead of time and keep in the fridge, covered, for up to seven days. This is perfect as a base for a pasta sauce. You can also serve it with steamed vegetables or reduce it slightly and use as a topping for pizza.

1   Put the tomatoes in a large saucepan over a medium heat.

2   Add the olive oil, oregano, bay leaves, garlic and thyme sprigs. Bring to a boil then reduce to a low-medium heat. Simmer gently for at least 30 minutes, or longer if you can, to bring all the flavours out.

3   Remove the bay leaves and thyme sprigs and season to taste. Either crush with a potato masher, or blend for a very smooth texture. Season to taste.

PONDICHERRY LENTIL SOUP

Serves 2
Preparation 1 hour

Ingredients
1 tbsp non-
hydrogenated
margarine
½ large onion, sliced
1 celery stalk, finely
chopped
100g red lentils
500ml chicken stock
salt and freshly
ground black pepper
1 tsp ground cumin

Lentils are high in nutritional value: they contain phosphorus for nerve function, iron to prevent anaemia, and magnesium for your general well-being. You will love this hearty soup!

1 In a large saucepan, heat the margarine over low heat, add the sliced onion and cook very gently until browned.

2 Add the celery and sauté for 10 minutes.

3 Add the lentils and sauté for 2 minutes, over low heat. Add the chicken stock.

4 Leave to simmer for 20-30 minutes, or until the lentils are just tender. Keep a close eye on them, because they can become mushy if overcooked.

5 Season to taste with the salt, pepper and cumin.

RED CABBAGE GAZPACHO

Serves 4
Preparation 25 min

Ingredients
¼ average-sized
red cabbage
1 Granny Smith
or Bramley apple
few drops lemon
juice
250ml apple juice
salt and freshly
ground black pepper
100ml light sour
cream
1-2 pinches ground
cinnamon

Here is a great recipe to enjoy as a light lunch on a hot day or when you are just looking for a light starter. Cabbages are an amazing source of fibre, vitamin C, potent antioxidants and sulphur. The red version of any vegetable or fruit means that it's even more charged with antioxidants (notably, beta-carotenes).

1   Wash, pat dry and slice the red cabbage.

2   Peel and core the apple and slice thinly, reserving one-quarter. (Squeeze a few drops of lemon juice over this to prevent it from going brown.)

3   Put the red cabbage, the three-quarters of the apple and the apple juice in a blender. To start with, just pulse to make sure the cabbage and the apple are chopped up evenly. Then, blend until everything is very finely chopped – the finer the better.

4   Strain through a fine-mesh sieve and season with salt and pepper.

5   In the meantime beat the cream until you have a foamy texture and add the cinnamon.

6   Mix the cream gently with the blended red cabbage, then add a last twist of pepper and a pinch of salt.

7   Dice the reserved apple, scatter over the gazpacho and enjoy!

SPLIT-PEA SOUP

Serves 2
Preparation 40 min,
plus soaking time

Ingredients
1 carrot
½ onion
1 garlic clove
½ courgette
olive oil
150g dried split
peas, soaked for 30
minutes to 1 hour
500ml chicken stock
½ sprig thyme
1 bay leaf
salt and freshly
ground black
pepper, to taste
a little fat-free
sour cream

1   Peel the carrot, onion and garlic, and cut the ends off the courgette.

2   Dice all the vegetables, keeping the garlic clove whole.

3   In a large pan, heat a little olive oil and add the diced vegetables along with the garlic. Cook for few minutes.

4   Drain the split peas and add them with the chicken stock, thyme and bay leaf.

5   Bring to the boil and season with salt and pepper.

6   Reduce the heat and simmer for 30-45 minutes.

7   When the vegetables are fork-tender, remove the thyme and bay leaf, and blend the soup with a hand-held blender.

8   Serve in individual bowls with 1 tsp sour cream per bowl.

BOK CHOY
WITH PRAWNS

Serves 4
Preparation 20 min,
plus 30 min

Ingredients
225g small prawns,
fresh or frozen
2 tbsp canola oil
2 heads of bok choy
(pak choi, or Chinese
cabbage)
1 apple, peeled
and diced
1 tbsp sesame
seeds
juice ½ lemon
fresh coriander or
chives, to garnish

For the vinaigrette
1 quantity
Soyannaise (p. 81)
1 slice fresh,
peeled ginger, finely
chopped; or 1 pinch
ground ginger
salt and freshly
ground black pepper

The sesame seeds in this dish increase
its calcium content.

1   Defrost the prawns, if using frozen.
Sauté in the canola oil until fully cooked.

2   Rinse the bok choy leaves and pat dry.
Slice and place in a salad bowl.

3   Add the prawns, apple and sesame
seeds.

4   Sprinkle over the lemon juice.

5   Make the vinaigrette by mixing together
all the ingredients. Add to the bowl and mix
well.

6   Leave for 30 minutes so that the lemon
starts 'cooking' the bok choy leaves.

7   Chop the coriander leaves or chives
and sprinkle over the salad before serving.

CHICORY BOATS WITH SMOKED SALMON

Serves 2 or more
Preparation 10 min

Ingredients
1 head chicory
2 tsp cream cheese per leaf (cow's milk, sheep's milk or vegan)
around ½ slice smoked salmon per leaf
1 small jar lump-fish roe, orange or black
dill, to garnish

Chicory (or Belgian endive) can be served cooked or raw. It's rich in kaempferol – a powerful antioxidant which reduces the risks of cancer in general, and also has a beneficial effect on some specific cancers. Chicory has also been shown to reduce the risk of cardiovascular disease. This delightful and nutritious dish is quick and easy to prepare and makes a lovely appetiser. Adjust the quantities depending on how many you are serving.

1   Wash and dry the chicory leaves. Spoon 2 tsp cream cheese onto each leaf.

2   Using scissors, chop the smoked salmon into fine strips over the cream cheese.

3   Top each 'boat' with a scant ½ tsp lump-fish roe.

4   Garnish with dill and serve chilled, as an appetiser.

CABBAGE BLINIS

Serves 4
Preparation 30 min

Ingredients
1 tsp juniper berries
1 cabbage, sliced thinly
4 eggs
1 tsp polenta
salt and freshly ground black pepper
25g non-hydrogenated margarine

These blinis can be prepared in advance and warmed in the oven before serving. They also freeze very well. They make a delicious light meal with steamed fish or a fresh salad.

1   Toast the juniper berries for 1 minute in a non-stick frying pan. Leave to cool, then crush them.

2   Steam the cabbage for a few minutes – it should stay slightly crunchy. Leave to cool.

3   Beat the eggs with the polenta, salt and pepper. Add the cabbage and crushed juniper berries.

4   Melt the margarine in small pan. Form little pancakes with the batter and cook over a low heat for 5–10 minutes on each side.

RAW PAD THAI

Serves 4
Preparation 1 hour

Ingredients

For the sauce
250ml reduced-fat coconut milk
125g Almond Butter (p. 225)
1 tsp jalapeno or red chilli, finely chopped
1cm ginger, chopped
2 tbsp Nama Shoyu or low-sodium soy sauce
1 tsp red miso paste
1 garlic clove crushed
2 tsp lime juice
2 dates, chopped
½ tsp cayenne pepper

For the 'noodle' base
450g daikon (oriental radish), or courgettes, finely shredded
70g kale, finely shredded
½ red pepper, finely sliced
2 medium carrots, peeled and grated
1 spring onion, chopped on the diagonal
40 Thai basil leaves (or Italian basil)
few sprigs coriander, finely chopped

For the garnish
½ cucumber, finely sliced on the diagonal
mixed greens (lamb's lettuce, baby spinach, rocket), for serving (optional)
8-10 cherry tomatoes, halved
110g chopped Teriyaki almonds or peanuts

This colourful, alkalising dish is lovely on a warm summer's day. It's very forgiving: you can substitute other vegetables, as you prefer. Ideally, shred the daikon with a mandolin or spirooli vegetable slicer.

1   To prepare the sauce, place all the ingredients in a blender. Blend on high speed until creamy and smooth. Taste and adjust flavours if necessary.

2   Ten minutes or so before serving, place all of the prepared vegetables from the 'noodle' base into a large bowl and toss with the prepared sauce.

3   Prepare your garnish while the vegetables are marinating. Fan out three of the cucumber slices on the edge of each plate and, if using green leaves, use these to garnish the other side. Place the Pad Thai mixture in the centre and top with the tomatoes and almonds. Serve immediately.

ROASTED POTATOES AND ARTICHOKES

Serves 4
Preparation 45 min

Ingredients

4 tbsp olive oil
1 large onion, finely sliced
1 tsp sugar (optional)
4 red potatoes
200g artichoke hearts, cut into 4 (fresh or frozen)
200g fresh or frozen peas
1 garlic clove, crushed
6 thyme sprigs
salt
about 1 litre chicken stock

This tasty recipe is ideal served as a main vegetarian dish with a side of baked tomatoes or Stir-fried Tofu with Dijon Mustard (p. 78). Remember that artichoke is packed with antioxidants: it's a detoxifying powerhouse!

1   Heat 2 tbsp olive oil in a pan and cook the onion very gently until caramelised. You may add 1 tsp sugar if they start to look dry, as this encourages them to release more liquid.

2   In the meantime, parboil the potatoes (in their skin). Remove them before they are fully cooked – they should remain firm and inedible.

3   When the potatoes have cooled, remove their skins and cut into cubes.

4   Over a gentle heat, add the potato cubes to the caramelised onion in the pan and mix to combine. Add the artichoke hearts and peas.

5   Add the rest of the olive oil to the mixture. Add the garlic and thyme and season lightly with salt (remember that the chicken stock already contains salt).

6   As soon as there is no more liquid in the pan, add the chicken stock, a little at a time. There's no need to soak the vegetables, but keep them moist. You may not use all the stock.

7   When the potatoes are fork-tender, remove the pan from the heat and serve hot.

SPAGHETTI SQUASH WITH MUSHROOMS

Serves 2
Preparation 45 min

Ingredients

1 spaghetti squash, halved lengthwise, seeds removed
2½ tbsp olive oil
250g mushrooms, such as chestnut or button, sliced
1 garlic clove, crushed
salt and freshly ground black pepper
a little grated Swiss cheese or soy cheese

It's worth trying to source spaghetti squash for this tasty low-carb dish. If you have any leftover cooked squash, it can be frozen and used in other recipes. It's delicious as a gratin, mixed with ingredients such as tomatoes or bacon.

1   In a large saucepan, place one half of the squash, flesh side down. Cover with water and bring to a boil.

2   Cover and simmer for 20 minutes.

3   In the meantime, heat the olive oil in a pan and sauté the mushrooms with some salt until tender and brown, and all the juices have evaporated. Add the garlic.

4   When the spaghetti squash is fork-tender, remove from the pan and let it cool. Place the second half of the squash in the same saucepan and cook in the same way.

5   Preheat the oven to 180°C/350°F/gas mark 4.

6   To make the 'spaghetti' strands, drag a fork across the flesh of the squash from end to end over a bowl (it will look like spaghetti). Save the shells.

7   Add the mushrooms to the squash flesh and season with salt and pepper.

8   Fill each shell with half the mixture and sprinkle with grated cheese.

9   Transfer the spaghetti squash to the oven and bake for 20 minutes until nicely browned. Check regularly after 12 minutes, as oven temperatures can vary so much.

SAUTÉED BABY BROAD BEANS

Serves 2
Preparation
20-30 min

Ingredients
1 tbsp olive oil
½ onion, peeled and finely sliced
½ red pepper, diced
1½ tomatoes, diced
1 spring onion, finely chopped
200g baby broad beans (if they are very young, keep them in their pods)
salt and freshly ground black pepper
50g asparagus spears, fresh or frozen
50g peas, fresh or frozen

Broad beans have been grown since prehistory – in fact, they're the oldest crop known to man. They contain vitamins A, B and E, as well as minerals such as calcium, copper, iron, magnesium and potassium.

1   Heat the oil in a frying pan over medium heat, add the onion and sweat it until it is translucent but not brown.

2   Add the pepper, tomatoes (with their juices) and spring onion. Stir well and bring to a simmer for 5 minutes.

3   If using very young broad beans in their pods, rinse, top and tail the pods, and chop them up in little segments. Otherwise, add the beans to the pan, season and stir.

4   Halfway through cooking, stir in the asparagus spears and the peas.

5   Cook for 10 minutes. Enjoy immediately!

VEGETARIAN BURGERS

Serves 2-4
Preparation 30 min,
plus 1 hour cooking

Ingredients
2 carrots, grated
2 celery sticks,
grated
2 courgettes, grated
1 small onion or
2 shallots, finely
choppod
480g sprouted
soybeans or
chickpeas (p. 194)
40g flour of your
choice: wheat, corn,
rioc, chickpea or
sweet chestnut
flour; potato starch
(potato flour)
handful of parsley
and chives, finely
chopped
pinch of curry
powder
2 tsp balsamic
vinegar
1–2 tbsp olive oil

I have not specified a size for the burgers –
it's up to you to decide. If you don't use
up all the mixture, you can cover it and
store in the fridge for 2–3 days. You can
also freeze any leftovers and reheat in a
non-stick frying pan.

1   Combine all the ingredients in a large
bowl and mix well.

2   Make burgers from the mixture,
according to the size you prefer. Flatten
them and transfer to a tray lined with
baking paper.

3   Bake for 1 hour at 100°C/225°F/gas
mark ¼.

4   Enjoy with a fresh salad for a delicious,
vegetarian meal.

MOCK MASH

Serves 2
Preparation 15 min

Ingredients
½ cauliflower
1 tbsp butter or
cheese spread, such
as Laughing Cow
salt and freshly
ground pepper,
to taste
nutmeg (optional)

Mock Mash is made not with potato or carrot, but with cauliflower and cheese. This is a true delight! Don't hesitate to make extra because it freezes very well.

1   Steam the cauliflower until it can be easily mashed with a fork.

2   Place in a bowl and mash with butter or cheese spread, salt, pepper and nutmeg, if liked.

CHICKEN PICCATA

Serves 2
Preparation 30 min

Ingredients
1 lemon
salt and freshly
ground black pepper
2 chicken breasts
60ml olive oil
25g non-
hydrogenated
margarine
70g mushrooms,
thinly sliced
½ garlic clove,
finely chopped
40g organic
wholewheat flour
60ml chicken stock
50ml white wine
1 tbsp capers
1 tbsp sugar

1   Peel the lemon with a sharp knife and remove the membranes. Cut it into pieces, reserving all the juice.

2   Season the chicken breasts. Heat a frying pan and add half the olive oil. Brown the chicken breasts over a medium-high heat for 3–5 minutes on each side. Remove from the pan, set aside and keep warm.

3   Add the margarine and remaining olive oil to the hot frying pan. Sauté the mushrooms for approximately 2 minutes.

4   Add the garlic and flour, then slowly add the chicken stock. Stir well and bring to a boil.

5   Add the lemon and its juice, the white wine, capers, sugar and some salt and pepper. Simmer for a few minutes and let the sauce reduce a little.

6   Pour the sauce over the chicken and serve hot with steamed green beans.

BEEF SPRING ROLLS

Serves 4
Preparation 60 min

Ingredients
2 tbsp olive oil
2 onions, finely
sliced
1 tsp sugar
(optional)
500g beef mince
1 tsp cumin
½ bunch coriander,
chopped
salt and freshly
ground black pepper
1 pack of rice wraps
(about 500g)
1 tbsp canola oil
salad greens and
1 bunch of mint,
to serve
chilli dipping sauce,
to serve (optional)

I like to use two different oils in this Asian dish. Why? Because olive oil has the strong flavour of Provence, whereas canola oil has very little impact on the final taste. If you prefer, you can cook the entire recipe in one oil, of your choice.

1   Heat the olive oil in a pan and add the onions. Cook very gently over a low heat, until caramelised. You can add 1 tsp sugar if they start to look dry, as this encourages them to release more liquid.

2   Add the mince and cook for 15 minutes, stirring to break it up. Add the cumin and chopped coriander, and season with salt and pepper.

3   Set aside and let the meat cool down before filling the rice wraps.

4   Place one wrap on each of 4 plates. Spoon the meat onto the wrap and roll it up like a spring roll, tucking in the ends. Repeat with the remaining wraps.

5   Heat the canola oil in another pan and fry the spring rolls until golden brown. Place them on a paper towel to absorb the excess oil.

6   Serve with salad greens, fresh mint and chilli dipping sauce, if wished.

CHILLI CON CARNE

Serves 4
Preparation 1 hour
30 min

Ingredients
3 tbsp canola oil
1 onion, chopped
1 garlic clove,
crushed
pinch of ground
cumin
1 red pepper,
washed, deseeded
and sliced into thin
strips
600g lean beef
mince
200g peeled,
chopped tomatoes
(from a tin is OK)
300g tinned red
kidney beans
500ml chicken stock
½-1 red chilli, finely
chopped (depending
on how hot you like
it!)
cayenne pepper
salt and freshly
ground black pepper

I always make this for at least four people as it freezes very well, and the flavours have a chance to develop if it's made ahead of time. Serve with brown rice, buckwheat or quinoa.

1   Heat the oil in a saucepan and sweat the onion and garlic with the cumin over medium heat, without browning.

2   Add the red pepper and cook gently until soft.

3   Add the mince and sauté over medium heat, until brown.

4   Add the tomatoes, the beans and the stock, then cook over a low heat for at least 1 hour. To fully develop the flavours, leave on a low simmer for up to 4 hours.

5   Add the chilli, cayenne pepper, salt and pepper. Serve hot.

Variations: Replace the beef with turkey mince or crumbled tofu.

PAPAYA GRANITA

Serves 1
Preparation 5 min

Ingredients
1 papaya
5 ice cubes
mint leaves,
to garnish

Papaya has been called the 'elixir of youth' because of the high levels of provitamin A, and vitamins C and E it contains, making it a potent source of antioxidants. Besides having a positive effect on the immune system these nutrients may guard against cancer and cardiovascular diseases. A small pleasure with multiple virtues! This is lovely as a summer dessert. You could easily substitute other fruit, such as melon or strawberries.

1   Cut the papaya in half.

2   Scrape the flesh from the skin and put it in a blender.

3   Add the ice cubes and whizz until you have a thick granita.

4   Pour into a martini glass or bowl and decorate with mint leaves. Enjoy right away!

PINEAPPLE CARPACCIO

Serves 1
Preparation 5 min

Ingredients
4 thin slices peeled, fresh pineapple
1 tsp orange flower water or vanilla extract

Whether it's hot or cold, I love making this quick dessert, which takes just 5 minutes. Pineapple is a superb source of fibre and vitamin C, and contains an enzyme which some say makes you lose weight since it 'burns' fat. Maybe, but this only seems to work in laboratories!

1   Arrange the pineapple on a small plate.

2   Sprinkle with orange flower water or vanilla extract before eating.

POACHED PEARS IN GOOSEBERRY JUICE

Serves 6
Preparation 45 min

Ingredients
750ml gooseberry juice

30g cornflour or potato flour

1 vanilla pod, split into two

zest of 1 lemon

20g granulated sugar

6 Bosc pears (or any variety you prefer), peeled

This simple, elegant dish is perfect for a dinner party. Replace the gooseberry juice with cranberry juice, if you prefer.

1   Blend 4 tbsp gooseberry juice with the cornflour until smooth. Add to a saucepan with remaining juice, vanilla pod, zest and sugar. Bring to boil over medium heat, stirring.

2   Cut the base of each pear so that they sit nicely in your saucepan.

3   Place the pears in the gooseberry juice and poach for 15–20 minutes over a low heat at a gentle simmer, until fork-tender.

4   Using a slotted spoon, transfer the pears to a plate. Raise the heat to high and cook the poaching liquid until it is reduced to a thick syrup.

5   Place the pears on individual serving dishes and drizzle with the syrup.

STRAWBERRY AND MELON SOUP

Serves 2
Preparation 20 min

Ingredients
1 small cantaloupe melon, halved

a little vanilla extract

1 tbsp agave nectar

5 strawberries

1   Using a melon baller, scoop out the melon to make balls for the garnish. Scoop out the remainder of the flesh.

2   Whizz the melon flesh in a blender until smooth. Add the vanilla extract and agave nectar and pulse.

3   Pour the soup into a large serving bowl, cover and refrigerate until ready to serve.

4   To serve, ladle into individual bowls.

5   Cut the strawberries into a variety of shapes, to decorate, and add them to the soup with the melon balls.

ÎLES FLOTTANTES

Serves 4
Preparation 45
min, plus overnight
refrigeration

Ingredients
500ml Almond Milk
(p. 137)
1 vanilla pod
4 medium eggs,
separated
6 tbsp agave syrup
1 tsp cornflour
pinch of salt
ground cinnamon,
to serve
toasted almond
flakes, to serve

This classic French dessert should be
prepared well in advance, as it needs at
least eight hours chilling time. If you prefer
not to use a microwave, make the quenelles
first and poach them in the vanilla-scented
milk for 7-10 minutes, at the end of step 2,
removing them before adding the egg yolks
and making the custard.

1   Place the almond milk in a saucepan.
Make a slit down the middle of the vanilla
pod and put it in the milk. Place a large mixing
bowl in the freezer.

2   Heat the milk until warm. Remove the
pod and scrape the seeds into the milk.

3   In a large mixing bowl, beat the egg yolks
with 2 tbsp agave syrup and cornflour. Add
half of the milk, slowly mixing well to prevent
the egg yolk curdling, then add the rest of the
milk and whisk well once more.

4   Keep the custard on a low heat for a
few minutes, whisking continuously, until it
thickens. Let it cool down. Refrigerate.

5   Pour the egg whites in the chilled
mixing bowl and add a pinch of salt.

6   Using a whisk, beat the whites, increasing
the speed progressively. Once the egg whites
are firm with soft peaks, gradually add 4 tbsp
agave syrup, and continue whisking until stiff.

7   Using two spoons to shape them, form
medium, even quenelles and lay 4 on each
microwavable serving plate, spacing them
evenly. Cook in the microwave for 30 seconds
per plate of 4 quenelles, at 800W.

8   Serve in pretty cups: place 1 ladleful
of custard and 2 quenelles in each one.
Refrigerate for a minimum of 8 hours, or
overnight.

9   Sprinkle a pinch of cinnamon and some
toasted almond flakes on the top of each
serving. Serve very chilled.

YOUR WEIGHT-LOSS PROGRESS PAGE

WEEK 1

WEEK 2

WEEK 3

WEEK 4

WEEK 5

WEEK 6

WEEK 7

WEEK 8

WEEK 9

WEEK 10

WEEK 11

WEEK 12

WEEK 13

WEEK 14

WEEK 15

WEEK 16

WEEK 17

WEEK 18

WEEK 19

WEEK 20

THE END

Here we are! If you have reached this page it means that you've either:

- Read the entire book and followed the programme, *or*
- Skimmed through the pages to get to the conclusion quickly (piece of advice: go back to the introduction and take the time fully to immerse yourself in the programme, starting with the two weeks of DETOX), *or*
- Read the book in one go and are now planning when to start. Please, don't be overwhelmed; go back to the beginning and get started, one day at a time. (Just a hint: the right time is *now*!)

If you are in the first category of readers, take a moment to look back and see how much your lifestyle has changed since we started out on this journey. You should be lighter, feel more energetic and empowered with new knowledge in all aspects of your life: fitness, nutrition, stress-management, sleep-management, motivation and more.

Whenever you feel your old habits creep back into your life, don't hesitate to return to the beginning of this book and re-programme your mind and your life. There is no shame in that. The unhealthy habits were accumulated over years – decades, even – so there is always the possibility that we need to get back to the drawing board once in a while, to fully eradicate them.

I would love to hear from you about your victories, your struggles and the solutions you found within this programme; please let me know about your favourite recipes and your favourite tips. I would be delighted to feature you as a VIP BootCamper on my blog (myblog.lebootcamp.com) so that you can make use of your success story by inspiring others. If you are game, drop me an email at valerie@valerieorsoni.com. Don't hesitate to share your journey via a blog right from the start – this will help others jump on the healthy-lifestyle bandwagon along with you.

In the meantime, I wish you an amazing life!

VALÉRIE ORSONI

REFERENCES

ALKALINE DIET

Ströhle A, Hahn A, Sebastian A. Estimation of the diet-dependent net acid load in 229 worldwide historically studied hunter-gatherer societies. *American Journal of Clinical Nutrition*. 2010;91(2):406–412.

Sebastian A, Frassetto LA, Sellmeyer DE, Merriam RL, Morris RC., Jr. Estimation of the net acid load of the diet of ancestral preagricultural Homo sapiens and their hominid ancestors. *American Journal of Clinical Nutrition*. 2002; 76(6): 1308–1316.

Frassetto L, Morris, Jr. R.C. RC, Jr., Sellmeyer DE, Todd K, Sebastian A. Diet, evolution and aging – the pathophysiologic effects of the post-agricultural inversion of the potassium-to-sodium and base-to-chloride ratios in the human diet. *European Journal of Nutrition*. 2001; 40(5): 200–213.

Reddy ST, Wang CY, Sakhaee K, Brinkley L, Pak CY. Effect of low-carbohydrate high-protein diets on acid-base balance, stone-forming propensity and calcium metabolism. *American Journal of Kidney Diseases*.

2002; 40(2): 265–274.
Dawson-Hughes B, Harris SS, Palermo NJ, Castaneda-Sceppa C, Rasmussen HM, Dallal GE. Treatment with potassium bicarbonate lowers calcium excretion and bone resorption in older men and women. *Journal of Clinical Endocrinology and Metabolism*. 2009; 94(1): 96–102.

Dawson-Hughes B, Harris SS, Ceglin I. Alkaline diets favor lean tissue mass in older adults. *American Journal of Clinical Nutrition*. 2008; 87(3): 662–665.

DETOX

Dodes, JE. The amalgam controversy. An evidence-based analysis. *J Am Dent Assoc*. 2001; 132: 348–356.

Kotkas LJ. Spontaneous passage of gallstones. *Journal of the Royal Society of Medicine* (Royal Society of Medicine Press). 1985.

Eaton DC, et al. Renal functions, anatomy, and basic processes. In: Eaton DC, et al. Vander's Renal Physiology. 7th ed. New York, N.Y.: The McGraw-Hill Companies; 2009.

Position of the American Dietetic Association: Food and nutrition misinformation. *Journal of the American Dietetic Association*. 2006; 106: 601–607.

Duyff RL. Healthful eating: The basics. In: Duyff RL. *American Dietetic Association Complete Food and Nutrition Guide*. 3rd ed. Hoboken, N.J.: John Wiley & Sons; 2006: 48.

Madhus K, Strommc A. Increased excretion of Cs-137 in humans by Prussian blue. *Zeitschrift für Naturforschung* 1968; 233b: 391–3.

Nesterenko VB, Nesterenko AV, Babenko VI, Yerkovich TV, Babenko IV. Reducing the 137Cs load in the organism of 'Chernobyl' children with apple-pectin. SMW 2004;134: 24–7.

GLYCAEMIC INDEX AND GLYCAEMIC LOAD

Foster-Powell K, Holt SH, Brand-Miller JC. International table of glycemic index and glycemic load values: 2002. *Am J Clin Nutr*. 2002; 76: 5–56.

Oregon State University works reviewed by Simin Liu, M.D., M.S., M.P.H., Sc.D. Professor and Director, Program on Genomics and Nutrition, Professor of Epidemiology and Medicine, UCLA School of Public Health.

University of Sydney: http://www.glycemicindex.com

YEAST CONNECTION

Crook, WG. The Yeast Connection Handbook. Jackson, Tennessee: Professional Books, Inc.; 2002. Crook, WG, Cass H.

The Yeast Connection and Women's Health. Jackson, Tennessee: Professional Books, Inc.; 2003

Nobaek S, Johansson M-L, Molin G, et al. Alteration of intestinal microflora is associated with reduction in abdominal bloating and pain in patients with irritable bowel syndrome. *Am J Gastroenterol.* 2000; 95: 1231–1238.

Elmer GW, Surawicz CM, McFarland LV. Biotherapeutic agents. A neglected modality for the treatment and prevention of selected intestinal and vaginal infections. *JAMA.* 1996;275:870-876.

Rembacken BJ, Snelling AM, Hawkey PM, et al. Non-pathogenic *Escherichia coli* versus mesalazine for the treatment of ulcerative colitis: a randomised trial. *Lancet.* 1999; 354: 635–639.

Majamaa H, Isolauri E. Probiotics: a novel approach in the management of food allergy. *J Allergy Clin Immunol.* 1997;99:179–185.

Tubelius P, Stan V, Zachrisson A, et al. Increasing work-place healthiness with the probiotic Lactobacillus reuteri: A randomised, double-blind placebo-controlled study. *Environ Health.* 2005 Nov 7.

Guglielmetti S, Mora D, Gschwender M, Popp K. Randomised clinical trial: Bifidobacterium bifidum MIMBb75 significantly alleviates irritable bowel syndrome and improves quality of life – a double-blind, placebo-controlled study. *Aliment Pharmacol Ther.* 2011; 33(10): 1123-1132.

INDEX

THANK YOU

The THANK YOU pages are always my favourite in any book. They are usually the first ones I read! I simply love seeing how much of a village it takes to produce a comprehensive book like this one. If it were me, I would place them at the beginning!

Anyway, this is where I get to thank all the people who have made this book a reality.

I am going to start with two ladies – Sara Hecht and Selina Prager – who have edited my text since day one. This is truly an international team: I'm from Corsica, Sara is from Australia and Selina is a South-African Londoner. One after the other, they have spent countless hours making sure my words are well chosen and the concepts clearly explained. For your time, for your dedication, and for the impressive end result, I thank you from the bottom of my heart!

To my team at LeBootCamp, Gwénaëlle Beau and Marion Bodin: thank you for answering my urgent requests for new recipes and new menus with wild ingredients in the blink of an eye.

To Philippe Gellman, Erik Dupontreué, and Mathieu Fussman: thank you for believing in me and sharing this amazing adventure with me. I am forever grateful that fate made our paths cross.

To Laura Zuili, my French agent, who started the journey with Heather Holden-Brown in London. Thank you for putting your faith in this project and for introducing me to this great publisher, Quadrille.

To the people at Quadrille: Jane O'Shea and Ed Griffiths – I am thrilled you decided to go along with my project. I cannot wait to see how all our forces combined can help us spread my concept of healthy living around the world.

To Charlotte, whose amazing feedback, experience and contribution have helped shape up the book you have in your hand. Word by word, line by line, Charlotte has made sure my writings would be understandable to all. Charlotte, you took a gold nugget and chiselled it into a lovely jewel.

To David, whose clean design has helped present the message of this book with clarity and style.

To my Dad: thank you for all the research you have continued doing for this book, for insisting on some concepts before anybody else had really acknowledged how important they were. And I am thankful also for all the great recipes you have created for this book.

To my son: thank you for gracefully handling my 'absences' from your life as I was writing and rewriting chapter after chapter, then deleting them and starting from scratch. Seeing your happy smile, knowing that you were doing great in school and that you were going to get into Carnegie Mellon right before this book was published made the whole enterprise even more meaningful. In the process you also became vegetarian, but that's another story!

To the man in my life: thank you for making my life so sweet and light; for making sure I get what I need most to move ahead in life: love and fun.

To Mom: because you are there, every day, any time, wherever I am and for whatever I need. Thank you. You rock and you are my rock.

To all the BootCampers around the world, who have been with me for so many years. Thank you for your support and for sharing your success with me. Seeing you slim down in a healthy manner has been so rewarding!

Finally, thank you to my supportive bunch of friends: Danielle, with whom I practise my news fast every Friday; Paula, who introduced me to life in the Highlands in the 18th century – a great way to clear my mind when I was juggling with cups, grams and ounces; Isabelle, who repeatedly asked me, "How far along are you?", pushing me to write faster; Souhila, who was a great (and successful) guinea pig for the DETOX phase; Florence and her cool recipes; Claire and her constant happy mood; Heidi, who has discovered who I am, really; and Aaron, for taking really cool pictures of me.

PS: thank you to author Diana Gabaldon for keeping me awake at night every time a new book comes out and for pushing me to have a book launch event in Inverness! My publisher will love this!